To Kenny Stan,
with best wishes

John M Braithe

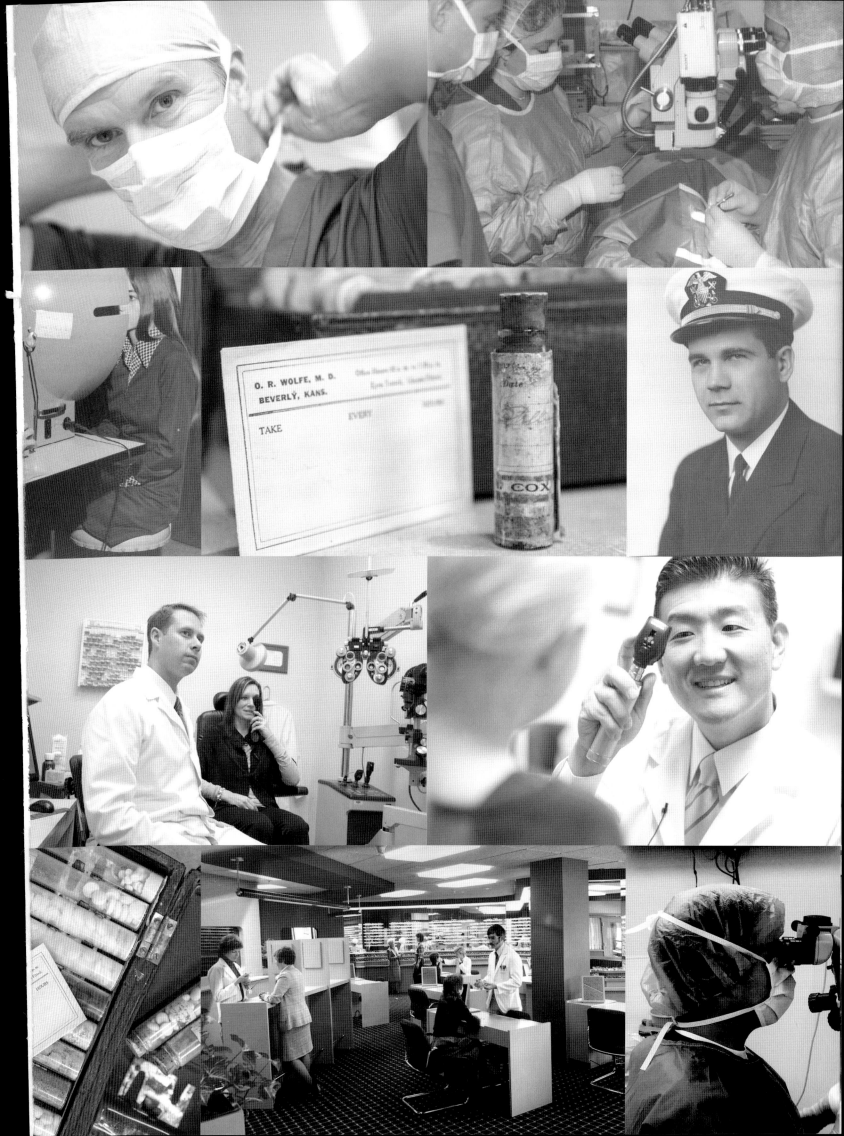

Wolfe Eye Clinic: A Century in Sight is published by
Business Publications Corporation Inc., an Iowa corporation.

Copyright © 2022 by Wolfe Eye Clinic:
A Century in Sight is a trademark of Wolfe Eye Clinic.

ISBN-13: 978-1-950790-04-3
Library of Congress Control Number: 2020923012
Business Publications Corporation, Des Moines, Iowa

Business Publications Corporation Inc.
The Depot at Fourth
100 4th Street
Des Moines, Iowa 50309
(515) 288-3336

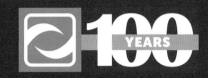

WOLFE EYE CLINIC

A Century in Sight

bpc

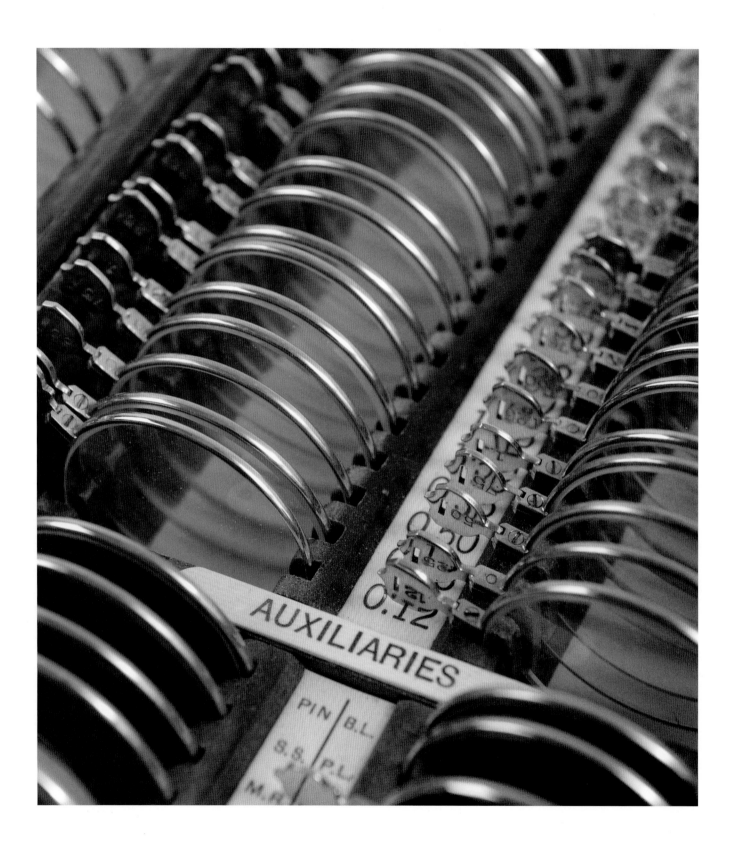

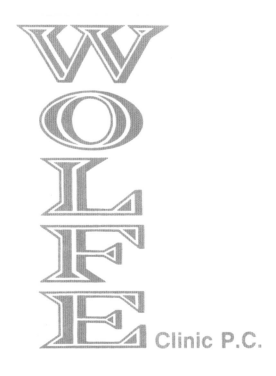

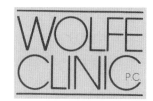

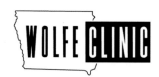

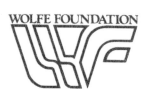

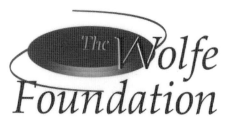

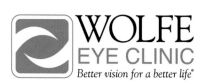

This book is dedicated
to the patients and friends of

WOLFE
EYE CLINIC

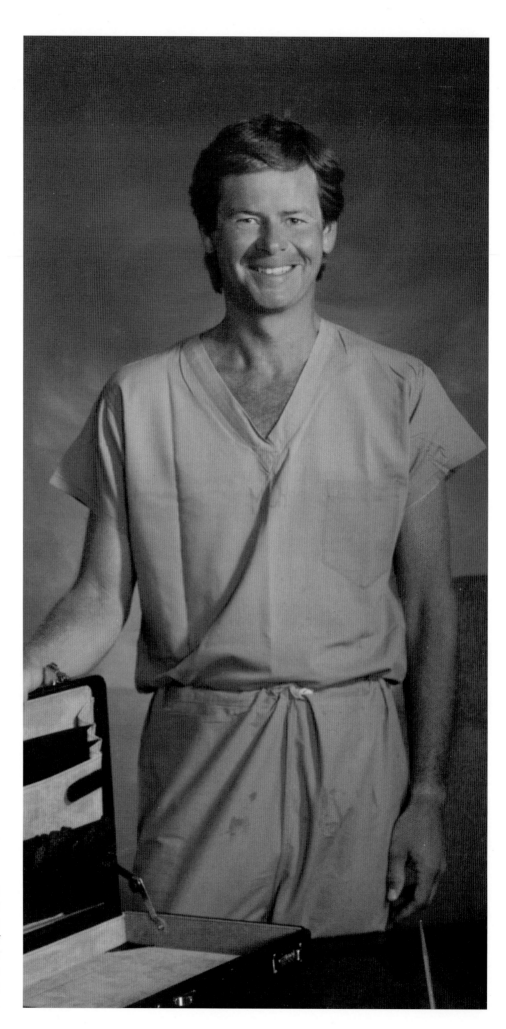

Dr. James Davison started at Wolfe Eye Clinic in 1980 and served as its president from 1995 to 2010. His many years of exceptional service and forward thinking help propel Wolfe Eye Clinic into the statewide organization it is today.

Wolfe Eye Clinic was founded in 1919 and this book, commissioned 100 years later, serves as a testament and history of the many years of quality eye treatment. We engaged Luke Manderfeld and the rest of the team at WriteBrain to help us write the book in an informal, friendly fashion and are very grateful for his successful "Iowa Style."

We have a lot to celebrate and be grateful for. Most practices or businesses don't survive 100 years. But Wolfe Eye Clinic has grown and flourished throughout its existence, evolving from one phase into the next. What began as a two-man practice grew into a family practice, then a group practice, then a small organization, then a larger one and is now emerging as an institution.

We have many people to thank, but our gratitude goes foremost to the patients and families who have trusted us with their care from the beginning. Our guiding principle has always been to think of them as family, and at all times and under all circumstances, provide the best-educated scientific advice and perform in their best interest.

Our gratitude extends to many more influential people and organizations. Particularly to Dr. Russell Watt and Dr. John Graether, two medical doctors who recognized the opportunities and satisfaction of joining the Wolfe family in practice. Thank you to the defacto chief recruiter, Dr. Otis D. Wolfe, who helped transition the family practice into the modern Wolfe Eye Clinic, and Dr. Graether, who was actively involved in recruiting doctors all

the way up to retirement as well. And thank you to Kevin Swartz, our recently retired CEO whose 27 years of advice and counsel was invaluable in building and sustaining the organization.

Wolfe Eye Clinic operates with the "Integrated Model," meaning surgeons and optometrists work together side-by-side to provide the best care. This practice was envisioned by the Wolfe family, supported by Russ and John and has been continued ever since. Through the cooperative, open and friendly professional relationship between optometrists and Wolfe surgeons, that model, which was for a long time thought of as renegade, is now common. It provides access to subspecialty medical and surgical care in offices across the state, closer to where patients live. We sincerely thank every one of our referring optometrists throughout Iowa and beyond for sustaining the immense support they've given us over the years. We also extend sincere gratitude to the many other doctors and health care professionals who turn to us for consultations and surgeries as well.

We offer sincere thanks to the many surgeons, optometrists, medical and surgical staff, executives and support staff who have served the patients of Wolfe

Eye Clinic since its inception. No matter the position, recruiting the best people has made it more likely to successfully attract and recruit more of the same. We thank them and their families for calling Iowa home and sharing their lives with us.

We have always been grateful for the ophthalmology and optometry industries and research partners who have continuously provided the most modern, ever-changing and wonderful medical and surgical devices and pharmacologic treatments. We are grateful to the many consultants, architects, builders, specialists and contractors who have helped shape our organization's corporate structure and facilities throughout the state. Our democratic governance has allowed us to create the best organization we could envision, including some of the best facilities imaginable. And importantly, the staff and equipment and facilities would not be needed if it weren't for the friendly and warm reception offered by host communities who invited us to join their medical communities in service. We thank all of them for their continued support.

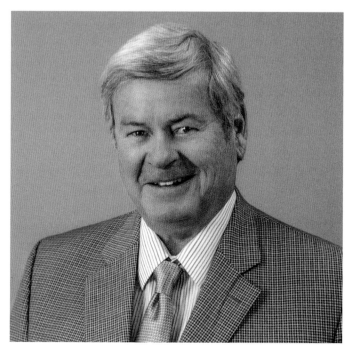

— James A. Davison, M.D., F.A.C.S.

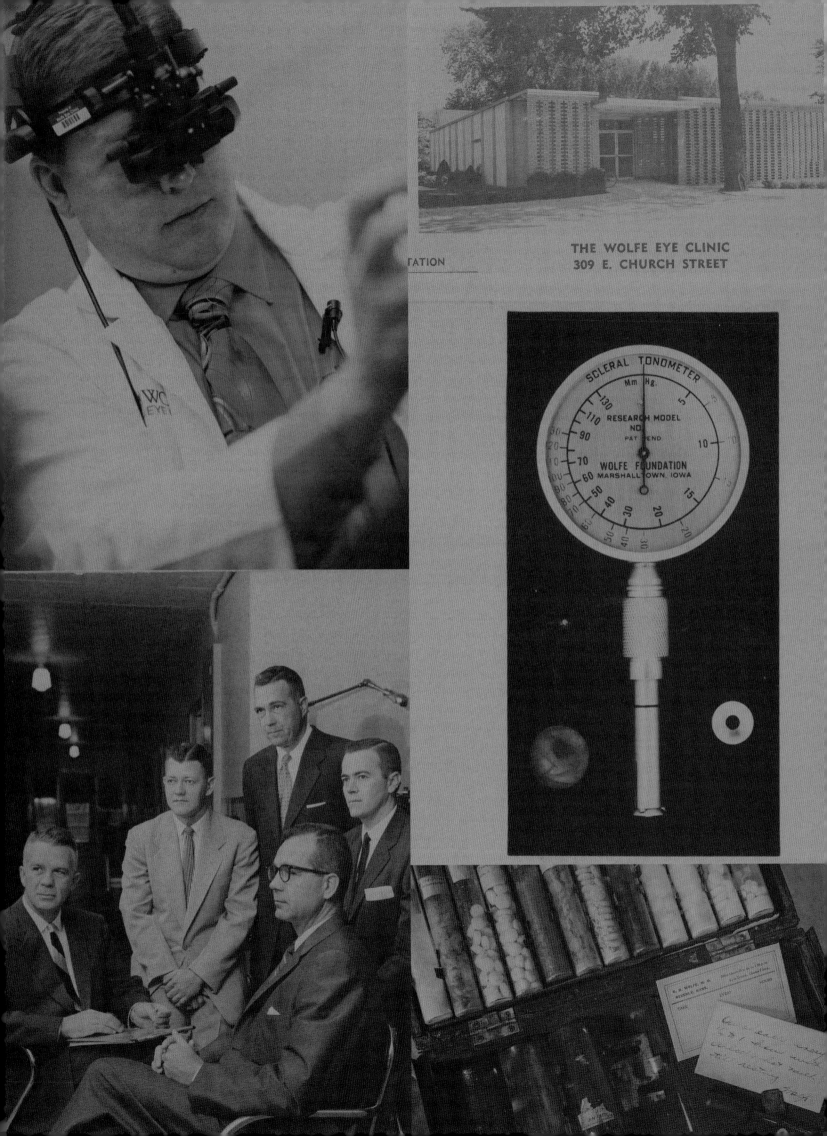

TATION

THE WOLFE EYE CLINIC
309 E. CHURCH STREET

SCLERAL TONOMETER

Mm Hg.

RESEARCH MODEL
NO.
PAT PEND

WOLFE FOUNDATION
MARSHALLTOWN, IOWA

HISTORY

100 Years of Eye Care Excellence

FOUNDED ON INNOVATION

Marshalltown was a city in the middle of everything. With a population totaling more than 15,000 in 1919 — making it one of the Iowa's largest at the time — Marshalltown had quickly become one of the state's epicenters for industry. Three railroads converged there, and it was also centrally located about 50 miles northeast of Des Moines. Business came from every direction, from Chicago to Omaha to St. Louis. This is where Dr. Otis Rudolph Wolfe planted the flag of his new business.

Wolfe was a brilliant, forward-thinking man, trained as a medical doctor in his home state of Kansas. According to Wolfe's unpublished autobiography, he found inspiration to become a doctor on the Sante Fe Railroad in Kansas City, Kansas, where he worked while in medical school at the University Medical College In Kansas City from 1906 to 1910. The surgeon on duty was a mentor, and Wolfe found himself spending extra time in the surgeon's office reading medical books. But Wolfe's inspiration to become an eye doctor was a bit more personal.

During medical school, Wolfe picked up chronic conjunctivitis from an old infection, causing acute flare-ups, along with visual imbalance. During his sophomore year, he wrote that his eyes were so bad he couldn't study anything for weeks at a time, needing his friends to read to him. He received treatment from various eye specialists who tried to help him with his problem and began to educate him about other eye diseases.

"This probably was a chief factor in causing me to decide to be an eye doctor," Wolfe wrote. "This, along with thinking that perhaps I could work out a way to perhaps improve my own eye problem."

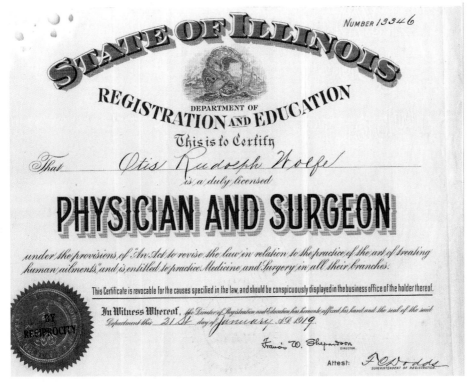

A certificate from the state of Illinois made out to Dr. Otis R. Wolfe showing his license as a physician and surgeon. Wolfe initially practiced in Illinois before coming to Iowa to start Wolfe Eye Clinic.

By 1918, Wolfe, 34 at the time, practiced both in Chicago and his home state of Kansas. In Chicago, he was training under two prominent eye, ear, nose and throat (EENT) doctors. Wolfe wanted to create his own business, something he could grow and innovate on his own. He began searching for practices to buy throughout the Midwest. He looked for towns where a business had potential while also providing a good place to raise a family. As legend has it, Wolfe picked up a map and circled Marshalltown, the place where the railroads and business met.

Wolfe packed up his bags and moved with his wife and three young sons. He bought a practice from Dr. Fred Lierle and partnered with fellow physician Dr. Frederick Wahrer to set up shop in February 1919 on the fourth floor of the Masonic Temple building in downtown Marshalltown.

Wolfe was a trained eye doctor. The clinic he purchased specialized in ophthalmology, a medical discipline focusing on eye care and surgery. Because of the clinic's central location, Wolfe and his partner treated patients all around the Midwest. Wolfe himself frequently traveled back to Chicago where he was referred patients in those early days, helping grow the clinic's regional client base.

Like today, innovation was an integral part of what made Wolfe Eye Clinic stand out. At the time, it was taboo for ophthalmologists to work with optometrists, who provided eye care but were not medical doctors. It was seen as a conflict of interest by the industry because of the disparities in their training. Whereas today many ophthalmologists

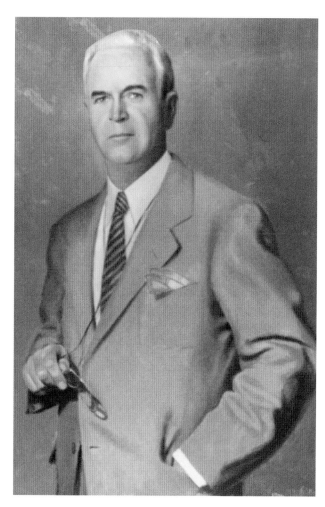

Dr. Otis Rudolph Wolfe

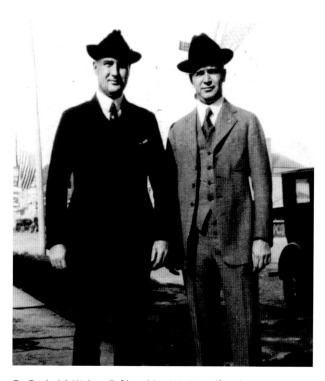

Dr. Frederick Wahrer (left) and Dr. Otis R. Wolfe, who went into business together in 1919 to create Wolfe Eye Clinic.

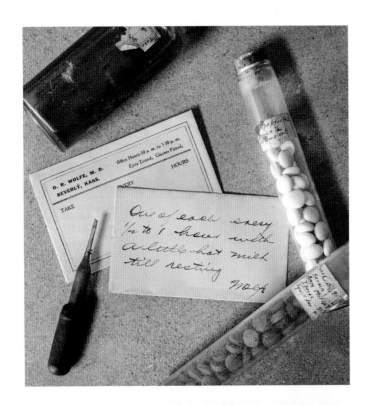

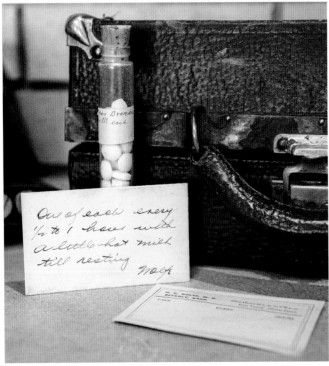

Notes from Dr. Otis R. Wolfe's briefcase, which include patient plans, schedules, medicine and more.

accept referrals from optometrists, that wasn't the case throughout the majority of the 20th century.

A common practice involving general practitioners and surgical specialists back in the day was "fee splitting," which meant family medical doctors referred patients to surgeons and might actually assist them in surgery or take a share of the surgical fee. According to notes from Wolfe's son, Dr. Otis D. Wolfe, his father wasn't interested in playing that game. Otis R. wanted to reach other locations around the state because for him, it was important to provide top-quality care to as many people as possible.

"Dr. Otis R. Wolfe claimed that he deplored the fee splitting practice and reached a turning point when a [general practitioner] came to him and said, 'French and Cobb gave me 50% for my patients. How much will you give me?'" Otis D. wrote. "He vowed to quit that practice and would turn to optometrists for support."

This alienated Otis R. from organized medicine. Otis D. wrote that his father received a warning about his behavior from the Judicial Council of the American Medical Association, but the practice had become a part of what endeared the clinic to generalists and their patients in Iowa and beyond.

Dr. Wolfe Is Interviewed on Trip to Spain

Barcelona is Up-to-Date But Not All of Spain

BY JOHN HYNEK

Having learned that Dr. Otis Wolfe of Marshalltown returned from his trip to Spain, your country editor said to himself, "Here is a friend who undoubtedly has observed things around him, and he ought to be interviewed," and so comes this story of how Spain and her people looked to the noted eye specialist.

Wheat in North Africa

Dr. Wolfe made the trip to Spain on a French liner which followed a course along the coast of Africa, and stopped at some points of interest, such as the city of Teneriff of the Canary Islands.

He had imagined Africa as mostly desert, and so was happily surprised to find north Africa a fine wheat country. There were no trees in Algiers, but there were fine trees in

Plow With Camel and Burro

The French are doing wonders in the way of progress in Morocco. One, however, sees strange sights. For instance on one side of a road, you may see a man plowing with a tractor, and on the other side you will see a native plowing with a team which consists of a camel and a small burro. Such an outfit hitched to a plow is not at all uncommon.

Even in Africa one sees motor cars. The roads are wonderful, and one travels at high speed in an auto on a fine road. Along the road there is a path for animals, and the autoist often meets a native riding a small burro on the path, the native often being a very large man on a burro which is not much larger than a dog.

The Arabs do not work. They are Nomads, and travel around, having some stock for grazing. The work is done by the Berbers.

Contrasts in Spain

On arriving in Spain Dr. Wolfe found great contrasts. For instance the city of Barcelona, where he spent most of his time, is as up-to-date and clean a city as one can find anywhere, but the rest of Spain is still living as people lived in medieval times. Even in Barcelona some modern customs are just beginning to creep in. But in

the next customer.

Barcelona is in the Catalonian part of Spain, and most of the people one sees are Catalans. Both the men and women are very handsome. They are proud of their ancient lineage.

Dr. Wolfe found the Catalans very democratic minded. He thinks that they want a republic instead of a monarchy. In fact, it is predicted in Spain that the present king will be the last one. The heir to the throne is a hemaphelac, or a victim of bleeding disease, and so will be physically unfit to rule. The people in this part of Spain do not want another king.

Need a Middle Class

Barcelona is the only city in Spain which has a middle class. In all other parts of the country there is no middle class. There are the aristocrats and the poor. This combination has resulted in the country being very backward. The Catalans are very ready to criticize the king and the government.

Women Just Starting

A woman is kept back everywhere in Spain, except in Barcelona in which city she is beginning to gain some recognition. In Barcelona one sees a few women office employes. Such a thing, however, is never seen elsewhere in Spain. In fact, in all other parts of Spain a woman never appears on the street without an escort. In Barcelona the women dress as they do in the United States, and so do the men. In fact, if one noticed the dress only, one would not know he were in a foreign country. The girls bob their hair and have the permanent wave just like they do in America.

The women expect to attain the vote soon, however. There is much activity for women's rights in Barcelona.

They Like America

The Catalans, Dr. Wolfe found, very friendly to America and great admirers of the United States. They love to talk about Uncle Sam, and they want their government and their business to adopt methods that are being used in the United States.

The Catalans also admire the English. The English language is being studied very much.

Bull Fight Surprised Him

Bull fights proved something entirely different from what Dr. Wolfe imagined they would be.

Andulasian bulls are used in the fight ring. Here in this country we have an idea that the fighting animals is a big bull. Your fighting bull, however, is a little animal. What

hospitals the country has are being operated by monks and nuns. Only the poor go to hospitals. Hence the hospital cases are charity cases. The monks and nuns are efficient in caring for the sick.

Dr. Wolfe found that in a hospital in Barcelona the monks and nuns were especially efficient. This hospital, however, was not all that was to be desired. For instance, there was no place for women patients in the eye department.

Dr. Barraquer a Genius

Dr. Wolfe, as is generally known, won national recognition by his success in performing the Barraquer method of operation for cataract on the eye. He went to Spain to work for a few weeks with Dr. Barraquer, the originator of this operation.

He found Dr. Barraquer, a genius and a prodigious worker. The Spaniard's father was an eye specialist, and the son undoubtedly inherited talents and received wonderful training. Dr. Barraquer's hobby is working in a machine shop. He has a modern machine shop at his home and employs a machinist. He gets his pleasure by working in this machine shop and he devotes most of his machine work to experiments in optical instruments.

Dr. Barraquer has several hospital rooms at his home for cases which require modern hospital care and special attention. He has had many noted patients, such as the Pope, the King of Spain, the Empress Eugenie of France, and other notables.

The hospital in Barcelona, while not having the one much needed women's department, however, was otherwise very up-to-date. In the eye clinic all the window lights were of green glass. There are many cases of eye trouble. The most numerous are cataract among the Catalans, and trachoma infection among the Andalusians.

The climate Dr. Wolfe found wonderful, and the country very beautiful in spring. Catalonia has no freezing weather even in the winter. Barcelona is a city of palms and eucaliptus trees.

A Lesson on Trees

We ought to learn a severe lesson from Spain regarding our forests. Dr. Wolfe found Spain a country of very few trees. On his trip to Madrid there was much soil erosion. Lands that once were productive and would be, were washed and cut up so that they were worthless.

It appears that in the fifteenth century a Spanish king cut up all of this forest to use for buildings. That country was once heavily forested.

A piece in the Tama News-Herald, dated in 1930, details Dr. Otis R. Wolfe's trip to Spain.

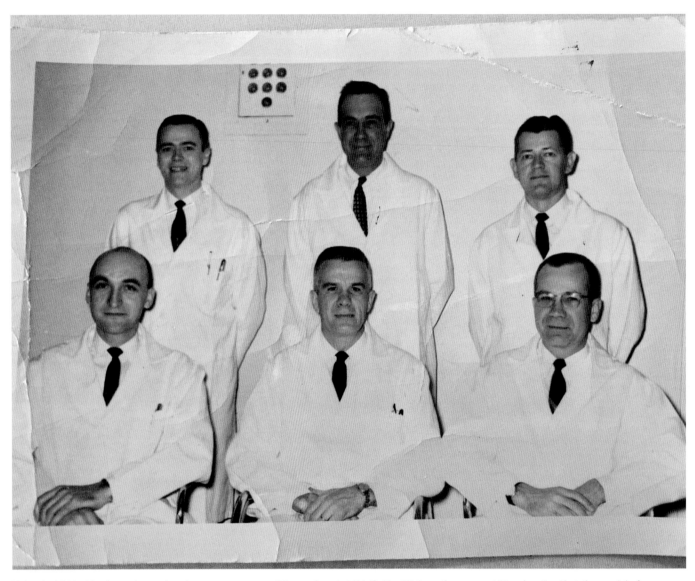

Taken in 1960, this photo shows that there were as many ODs employed at Wolfe Eye Clinic as there were MDs, showing that the model of partnership employed by Wolfe was unique in its kind. Front row: Russell Watt, Otis Wolfe and Russell Wolfe. Back row: Harry Rasdal, Henry Wolfe and Jerry Nesset.

Optometrists were not trained to perform surgery, so they could not assist during procedures but were more than happy to refer to an ophthalmologist they knew and trusted, especially if they knew their patients were getting top-notch care and would return to their practice after surgery.

In 1925, Otis R. again showcased his forward-thinking prowess. He had heard of a revolutionary cataract procedure performed in Spain by Dr. Ignacio Barraquer. Prior to this, most cataracts were removed using the extracapsular method. This new procedure was called intracapsular cataract extraction, a more effective method at the time because of its complete removal of the entire cataractous lens, ensuring the eye had no unremoved cataract substance and reducing postoperative inflammation, thus enabling faster recovery.

According to a newspaper article in 1925, Otis R. performed one of the first Barraquer method surgeries in Iowa. Some reports say it was one of the first in the United States. He was recognized in both the 1926 and 1928 eye, ear, nose and throat volumes of the Book of Practical Medicine.

"It is his work in removing cataract from the eye that has won him the most recognition," read an article in the Marshalltown Times-Republican. "Dr. Wolfe has followed the method of Dr. Barraquer, a noted Spanish specialist and has also discovered some new ideas on this operation."

Later that decade, Otis R. sailed by ocean-crossing steamer to Spain to learn more about the procedure from Barraquer himself — a trip that was detailed in a 1930 issue of the Tama News-Herald.

"Dr. Wolfe, as it is generally known, won national recognition by his success in performing the Barraquer method of operations for cataract on the eye," it read. "He went to Spain to work for a few weeks with Dr. Barraquer, the originator of this operation. He found Dr. Barraquer to be a genius and a prodigious worker."

Otis R. published his adaptation of the surgical technique and the results of his first 125 intracapsular cataract surgeries.

The innovative procedure combined with the unorthodox practice model of working with optometrists led to success for Otis R. Newspaper clippings in the late 1920s and 1930s

detailed successful surgeries completed on people from states including Illinois, New York, Texas, Missouri, North and South Dakota, and others.

A 1934 article in the Des Moines Tribune told the story of a 28-year-old South Dakota woman who had been mostly blind for years. She had just had twin babies, but could never distinctly see them. After being told she would have to remain completely blind for several years before being operated on, she found her way to Otis R., who restored her eyesight using the Barraquer method.

"I can't believe that I'm not dreaming," Mrs. L.N. Hare is quoted as saying. "It's so good to be able to see, and to look at things and recognize them, and to distinguish my friends by their faces instead of their voices. I think that I'm the happiest woman in the world."

Because of Marshalltown's geographic connectiveness to the rest of the country by way of the railroad, the clinic saw its best decade yet in the 1930s. Otis R. became the sole owner of the enterprise after buying out his partner Wahrer who had become ill, rendering him unable to practice. He named the clinic the Wolfe Cataract Clinic, giving more credence to his ground-breaking procedure. Otis R. found new ways to give back, too. He started the Wolfe Cataract Foundation in 1936, which helped fund indigent care and support of the community.

In just a few more years, more members of the Wolfe family joined the practice. And more innovation was on the horizon.

A FAMILY AFFAIR

Otis R. and his wife had four sons, Otis D., Russell, Henry and Paul. Paul was the youngest and the only son born in Marshalltown, just five months after the family arrived — the rest were born in Kansas. Throughout the 1930s, Otis D., Russell and Henry trained in various parts of eye care. Otis D. and Russell became ophthalmologists and Henry became an optometrist, with all three eventually joining their father in practice in Marshalltown.

When the United States joined World War II, all four sons joined the service. In February 1943, Paul was killed in action after a Nazi submarine sank his ship. The three other sons would eventually return and join their father in practice.

Wolfe Eye Clinic continued to thrive, albeit in controversial fashion. Otis R. further endeared himself to optometrists, and his cutting-edge cataract surgeries were gaining fame throughout the country. The name at the time, Wolfe Cataract Clinic, upset some in the industry. It implied that was all the clinic did.

"It sounded solicitous," Otis D. wrote in notes detailing the clinic's history. "It was. It also left the impression that that was the only thing the office did — cataracts."

But Otis R. liked to zig when others zagged, and business was booming. After the war, Otis D. joined his father in practice. Russell and Henry were recruited to join the family business a few years later.

The two surgeons Otis D. and Russell had quite different personalities. The oldest brother, Otis D., was a charismatic man, known for wit and looks. He was active in the field of medicine, being the head of a medical society in Des Moines. He was a highly skilled surgeon — and a passionate one at that.

"He was an excellent surgeon," said Dr. John Graether, who joined the clinic in 1962 and worked with the Wolfe family. "He was very, very skilled, and enjoyed surgery."

Russell was a good surgeon as well but had a more quiet and reserved personality. He worked hard, and enjoyed hunting and fishing. The two brothers worked cohesively and formed a business partnership with the

But Otis R. liked to zig when others zagged, and business was booming.

third brother, Henry, in the mid-1950s after Otis R. retired.

Henry had been with the clinic at the urging of his father since the conclusion of World War II. As an optometrist, Henry examined patients, testing their vision, fitting them with glasses and referring those needing surgery to his brothers. But as the business grew, Henry played a bigger role in the administrative side of the business.

Things continued to look up for Wolfe Eye Clinic in the 1950s. Soon enough, that growth led to the clinic's first hiring of physicians outside of the Wolfe family. Dr. Russell Watt was brought on in 1959, and became the first non-Wolfe family member ophthalmologist on staff. He was followed by Graether in 1962.

The eye surgeon quartet of the two Wolfe brothers and Watt and Graether launched an era of unprecedented growth for Wolfe Eye Clinic. They introduced new procedures to the area and continued the brand of top-quality care that would eventually define Wolfe Eye Clinic for 100 years.

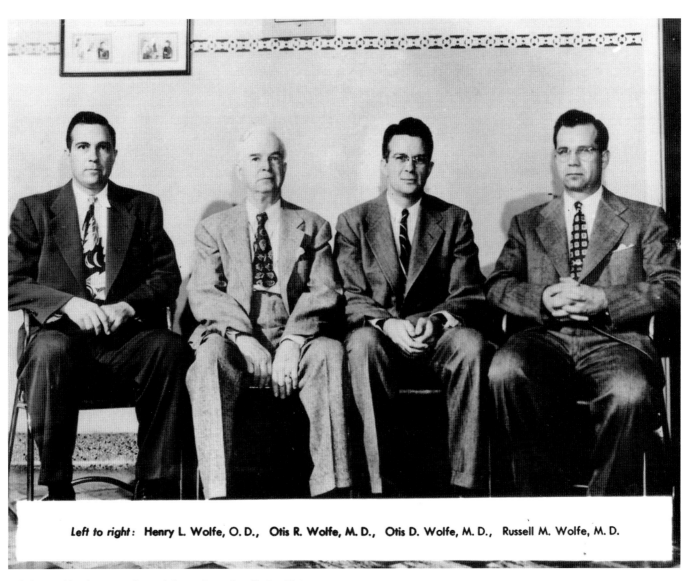

Left to right : Henry L. Wolfe, O. D., Otis R. Wolfe, M. D., Otis D. Wolfe, M. D., Russell M. Wolfe, M. D.

A father and his three sons formed the nucleus of Wolfe Eye Clinic.

CARRYING THE STANDARD

By 1950, Otis R. was becoming less and less involved in the business, particularly as his battle with colon cancer continued. He succumbed to the disease in 1954 in Rochester, Minnesota, and was memorialized by the editorial board at the Marshalltown Times-Republican.

"In the eye clinic that he established at Evangelical Hospital, and especially in his own work in children's eye diseases, Dr. Wolfe's work will live on after him — a goal that many men seek but few reach," the article read. Otis R.'s legacy continued through his sons and new ideas from new physicians.

Cataract surgeries were still the clinic's bread and butter, and Watt and Graether were outside-the-box thinkers as well and wanted to try new and better things. The hiring of Watt and Graether also helped soothe the long-standing animosity between the clinic and the ophthalmology profession, which was still uncomfortable with the organization's relationship with optometrists.

When Graether was recruited to join Wolfe Eye Clinic in 1962, he recognized its unique mindset right away. Other practices were more conservative, but these physicians were not. They were open to change, open to something new.

"This was an atmosphere where new ideas were acceptable and encouraged," Graether said. "In a lot of practices that was not the case. It was the strength of Wolfe Eye Clinic, and I recognized that, and it was one of the biggest reasons why I joined the clinic."

It was a perfect time to be open-minded. The ophthalmology profession was undergoing significant change, with new procedures being revolutionized and perfected all across the world. Just as technology was beginning to ramp up across all professions, so too were processes and procedures in ophthalmology.

Wolfe Eye Clinic was on the cutting edge of the changing times, performing a number of new surgeries in the 1960s, including corneal transplants, ocular microsurgery and xenon

arc photocoagulation, which was the first form of light therapy to treat retinal disease. At the turn of the decade, Dr. Russell Widner and Dr. Gilbert Harris joined, helping fuel more forward-thinking within the organization.

There was a friendly competitive edge around the office, and it pushed patient service to new levels. After operations, patients were often evaluated at dismissal by another physician in the clinic. That meant everyone's surgical work was being examined, right away after surgery and then weeks and months later in follow-up. They were always learning.

"Drs. Watt, Graether, Widner and Harris were the ones that really pushed this to the next level," said Kevin Swartz, CEO of Wolfe Eye Clinic. "Part of that was due to timing and what was happening in ophthalmology at the time. The organization has always been a cooperative group of forward-thinking people who tried to do things just a little bit better. Innovation came from the competitive nature of these guys."

A giant surgical breakthrough came in 1972, when Wolfe Eye Clinic was the first in Iowa and one of the first in the United States to perform small-incision phacoemulsification surgery, a

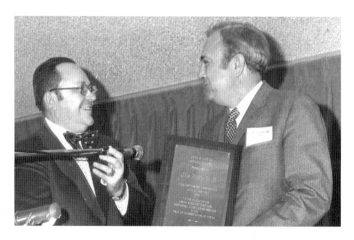

Dr. Henry Wolfe accepts the John E. Martin Annual Award from the Iowa Optometric Association, given to an "educator or vision scientist who has performed outstanding service in the field of conservation of vision."

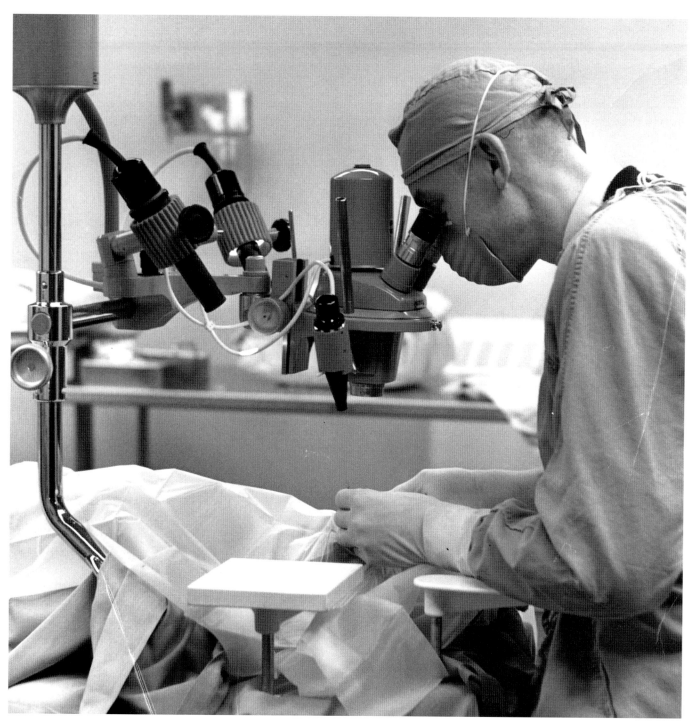

Dr. Russell Watt performs surgery using the Clinic's first operating microscope.

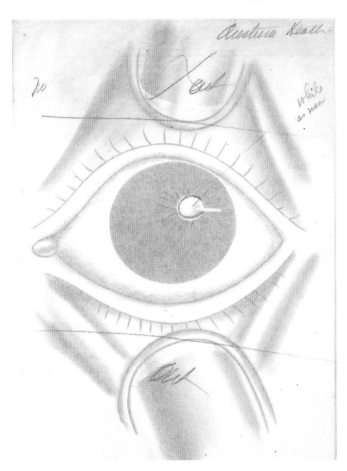

An early illustration showing a cataract and the rest of the eye.

less invasive and safer method of cataract surgery. Wolfe Eye Clinic purchased one of the first phacoemulsifiers — the tool used in the surgery — commercially available in the country.

Small-incision phacoemulsification was considered by many to be too risky at the time as surgeons were learning to apply new surgical techniques while using this new ultrasonic energy-vacuum needle machine. But Graether, who performed the first surgery, said Wolfe Eye Clinic didn't experience a lot of complications. The mixture of experience, skill and risk tolerance allowed the physicians to have an overwhelmingly low complication rate — around 2 to 3%, he said.

In 1975, Wolfe Eye Clinic performed the first intraocular lens implant surgery in Iowa, helping substantially grow its number of cataract patients. The procedure was crucial for the advancement of cataract care. Beforehand, surgeons completely removed the cataract, and patients were required to wear thick glasses that created very distracting visual distortions. Those distortions were eliminated because the plastic lens implants actually replaced the natural lens right inside the eye and thus restored the patient's natural vision.

By the early 1980s, new types of procedures were being performed almost every year, a reflection of Wolfe Eye Clinic's willingness to innovate and the changing of the industry at large. And Wolfe Eye Clinic continued to grow. It had moved into its own new building on the east side of downtown Marshalltown in 1961 and expanded that location in 1978, tripling its previous space, and added Dr. Michael Hill, an an ear, nose and throat surgical specialist.

But Wolfe Eye Clinic had yet to explode outside of its home city — something that would change in the next decade.

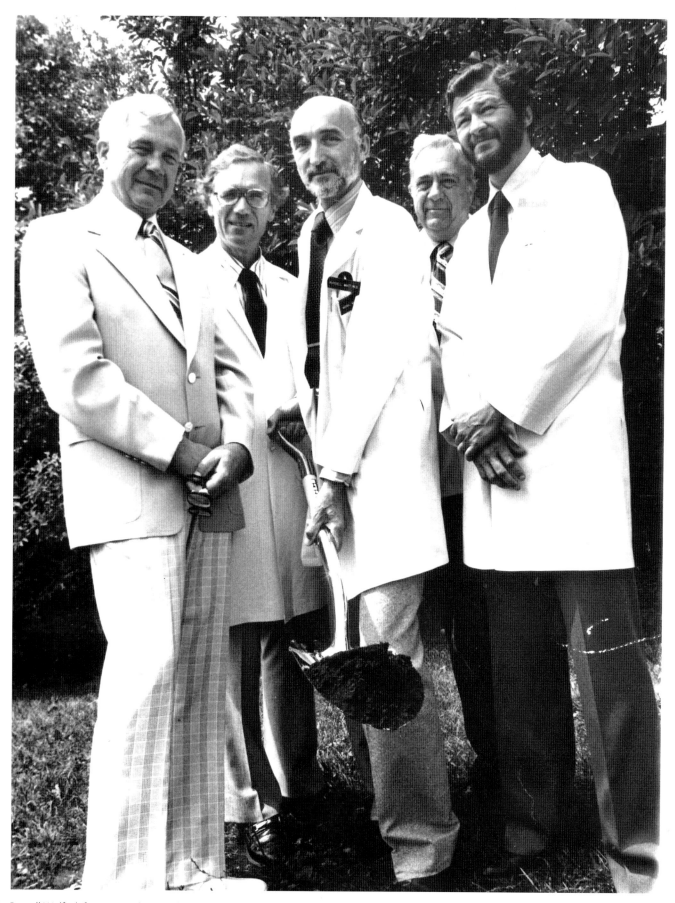

Dr. Russell Wolfe, left, poses with Drs. John Graether, Russell Watt, Henry Wolfe and Russell Widner during the groundbreaking ceremony for the new Marshalltown office addition in 1978.

STATEWIDE REACH

The call came out of the blue. It was fall 1981, and the person on the other end was Gov. Robert Ray's assistant. The wildly popular Ray wanted Graether to perform lens implant surgery to fix a cataract problem in his right eye.

Implant procedures were not as widespread as they are now. Other clinics deemed the surgery too risky — so much so that Graether said only about 10% of ophthalmologists in the country were doing the operation. But Wolfe Eye Clinic boasted skilled and forward-thinking surgeons who had already performed about 4,000 lens implants between them.

Ray would be the highest-profile case yet. On the day after Thanksgiving in 1981, Ray underwent the procedure. It took about 35 minutes, according to a Des Moines Register report, and the surgery was an overwhelming success.

"I performed his surgery on a Friday, and that weekend, there was a quarter-page picture of the governor in the Des Moines Register sitting in his office as if nothing had happened," Graether said with a laugh.

Wolfe Eye Clinic had been on the cutting edge throughout its entire history, but this surgery helped spread that message across Iowa and beyond. News about the procedure was supposed to stay quiet, but word quickly leaked out. Graether said more than 130 articles appeared in newspapers across the state. Ray was a popular guy, and every news organization tracked his progress.

"You couldn't buy the PR that resulted, it was ridiculous," Graether said. "It had a tremendous impact on the clinic's growth."

Ray's vision was perfect and two months later he wrote a letter of thanks to Graether.

"I just wanted to make sure that you know how deeply appreciative I am for what you have done for me," the governor wrote. "Please know that, in me, you have a strong advocate and grateful patient. Thank you

Wolfe Eye Clinic had been on the cutting edge throughout its entire history, but this surgery helped spread that message across Iowa and beyond.

and may you continue to bring brightness and happiness to many more."

The procedure on Ray marked the beginning of a new era for Wolfe Eye Clinic, which saw itself expand beyond its home in Marshalltown and reach new heights. All of the clinic's great physicians and their innovative procedures were put squarely on the map.

In 1984, Wolfe Eye Clinic opened its first location away from Marshalltown in rapidly growing West Des Moines. More terrific ophthalmologists had been brought on board, including Dr. James Davison in

1980. Davison has become one of the most highly regarded and requested surgeons in the Midwest, and he has been part of a number of new procedures and Iowa firsts at the clinic.

When Davison was looking for a place to work after a residency at the Mayo Clinic in Rochester, Minnesota, he noticed there was something different about Wolfe Eye Clinic — something intriguing.

Times-Republican

Central Iowa's Daily Newspaper

No. 281　　MARSHALLTOWN, IOWA, FRIDAY, NOVEMBER 27, 1981　　25 Cents

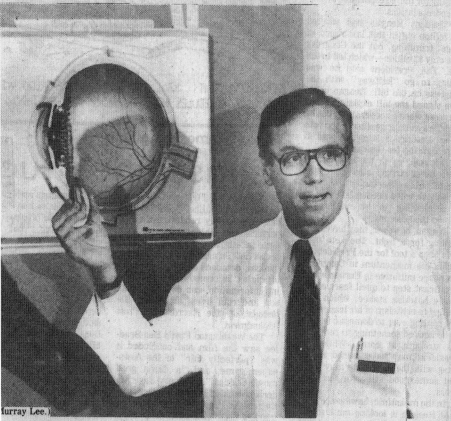

(Murray Lee.)

Y 'SMOOTH' — Dr. ...er, Wolfe Clinic ...t, explains the removal of a cataract from Iowa Gov. Robert Ray's eye Friday morning. Graether described the early morning surgery at Marshalltown Area Community Hospital as "very smooth" and without complications.

Governor's Eye Surgery Here Called Smooth

Iowa Gov. Robert Ray underwent cataract surgery Friday morning at Marshalltown Area Community Hospital and the procedure "went very smoothly" according to Dr. John Graether, ophthalmologic surgeon who performed the operation.

At a press conference Friday, Dr. Graether described the procedure as an "intraocular lens implant" in which the cataract - an eye lens which becomes opaque and interferes with vision - is surgically removed and replaced with an artifical lens made of a special plastic used in most hard contact lense

Dr. Graether said the surgery on the governor's right eye took about 35 minutes and is one of the most common procedures done by Wolfe Clinic surgeons. More than 4,000 such surgeries have been done in Marshalltown since Wolfe Clinic personnel began performing them in the spring of 1975.

Gov. Ray is expected to return home Saturday and will return to Marshalltown to be examined by Dr. Graether in a couple weeks and then in about a month to receive corrective lenses. The governor now wears glasses for reading purposes, and when he returns for his examination next month, Dr. Graether said he will prescribe a new pair of glasses primarily for reading.

The governor was accompanied by his wife, Billie, and an aide. Dr. Graether said Gov. Ray was "a very cooperative patient" and he didn't anticipate any complications following the surgery. The governor is expected to return to most normal activities in about two weeks.

Dr. John Graether explains the surgery he performed on Gov. Robert Ray, which was widely publicized at the time.

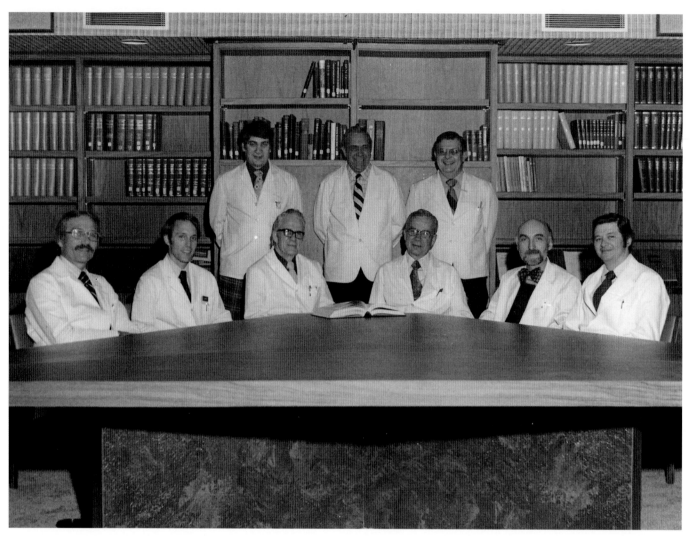

A 1974 photo of Wolfe Eye Clinic physicians in the library of the Marshalltown office. Sitting left to right, surgeons John Graether, Gilbert Harris, Otis Wolfe, Russell Wolfe, Russell Watt and Russell Widner. Standing from left to right, optometrists Jim Shuhart, Henry Wolfe and Doral Chapman.

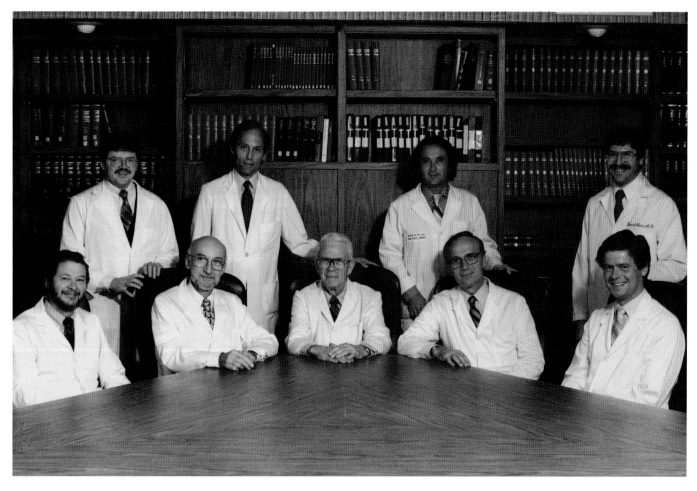

The 1984 Wolfe Eye Clinic Board of Directors. Seated from left to right: Russell Widner, Russell Watt, Otis Wolfe, John Graether and Jim Davison. Standing left to right: Norman Woodlief, Gilbert Harris, Micheal Hill and Daniel Blum.

"It was really impressive," Davison said. "I wanted to do something that would be interesting and fun and new, and here were these great guys in Iowa. They had this great model of working with optometrists, and they were doing great science. Nobody was doing the stuff they were doing. I could sense the culture of innovation and the desire to push each other to do better."

In 1986, a Fort Dodge location opened, followed by Cedar Falls in 1988, and Cedar Rapids in 1991. In 1997 the clinic finalized its merger with the three surgeons of Iowa Eye Care Physicians in Ames to create a new office there. Many of the physicians were traveling hundreds of miles a week to tend to patients in all parts of the state, part of the organization's long-standing dedication to providing the best care to as many individuals as possible. Kevin Swartz, a certified public accountant by training, joined the clinic in 1993 as its CEO, during the company's ascension. He brought systems accountability to the business. He was also a terrific recruiter and found excellent new surgeons who were placed in locations where their education and skills were needed. He facilitated placing Wolfe Eye Clinic outreach locations throughout Iowa, which allowed subspecialist surgeons to go into smaller cities to perform surgeries closer to patients' homes.

Many years later, Graether realized just how big of an impact these new locations had on the surrounding areas.

"We made sure that our outreach clinics were staffed by competent subspecialists on a rotational basis," Graether said. "So we brought a very high level of ophthalmic skill to rural areas that wouldn't have had them without that combination of our satellite offices plus the ability to rotate in subspecialists scheduled to provide that high

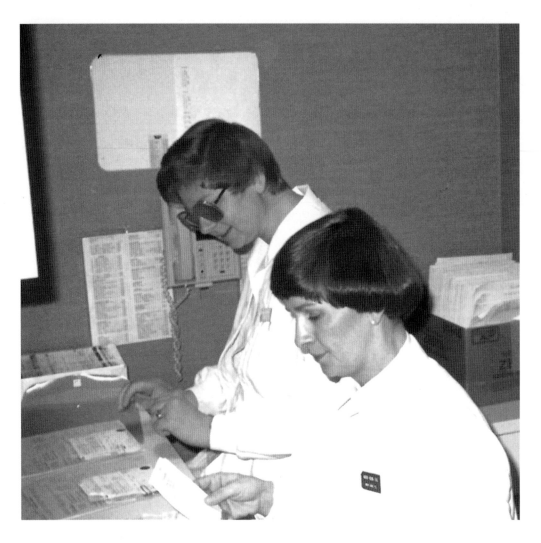

level specialty training in all of our environments."

Swartz noticed the impact, too. And patients were appreciative. Physicians who traveled to different locations were often booked out months in advance, validating the success of Wolfe Eye Clinic's burgeoning business model.

"You've got to grab opportunities," Swartz said. "Just like anything else in life. We needed to look at the next step and make sure that, for our patients, we were going to be able to give them the best answer and the best options available."

In those couple of decades, the Wolfe family phased out

of the business. Russell retired in 1978 and he and his wife moved to Horseshoe Bend, Arkansas. Henry retired to Texas after an agreement was reached between him, his brothers and other physician owners. Otis D. was the last Wolfe family member remaining when he retired in 1991. He was almost 80.

By 1992, Wolfe Eye Clinic had a staff of more than 100 people — nine of those were ophthalmologists, who served as owners in the business. The Wolfe family had been a part of the company for 72 years and were obviously integral in its rise to prominence.

In a 1991 Des Moines Register article covering his retirement, Otis D. said he had witnessed major advancements in eye surgery during his nearly 50-year career. New laser and surgical techniques were being performed every year. Well before his retirement, it was not uncommon for cataract patients to spend 10 days in the hospital after surgery.

"Now we can send them home the same day," he was quoted as saying in the article.

That was thanks to the brilliance of the Wolfe family and the many ophthalmologists who joined the family in practice.

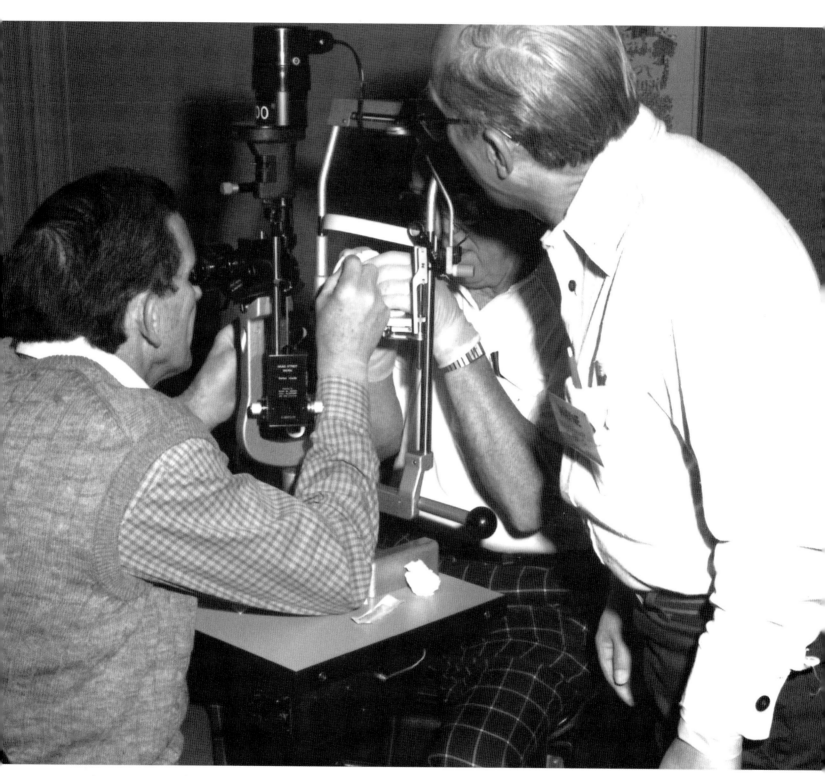

Above: Optometrists from all over Iowa were being trained in new techniques at Wolfe Eye Clinic.

Opposite page: Two Wolfe Eye Clinic team members look over paperwork.

SPECIALTY EYE CARE

The 1990s brought the rise of subspecialization in the medical field, and ophthalmology was included. Before the decade, most general ophthalmologists had a hand in everything from cataract to pediatrics to retina. But with more technology and improved procedures came the need for more expertise in specific subspecialized fields like cornea, glaucoma, cataract and refractive, pediatrics and strabismus, retina and oculofacial plastic surgery.

Wolfe Eye Clinic was also serving a bigger market — particularly the relatively densely populated Des Moines and central Iowa area — and thus needed to bring in more physicians to specialize in various procedures. The company had expanded throughout the state and began to perform more than cataract surgeries, which had been booming in numbers the previous decade.

Dr. David Saggau, currently in retina disease and surgery, joined Wolfe Eye Clinic during that critical transformation. He had completed a retinal fellowship in Cleveland before moving to Iowa in 1990. While he did a lot of retina work when coming on board, he was also involved in cataract, pediatric and more. Saggau was originally located in Marshalltown, but relocated to West Des Moines where there were more patients who needed specialty care. Physicians were being hired to address these specialty needs and give patients the best care possible.

"When I came in, we were kind of on the edge of that subspecialty transition," Saggau said. "It made for better care, and it was more efficient care. That wasn't just unique to ophthalmology. It's kind of weird to think that an eyeball, for the size it is, has so many little subspecialties, but it does. And they're all important."

Wolfe Eye Clinic quickly expanded into multiple subspecialties, including retina, LASIK — the first LASIK procedure was performed in 1996 — glaucoma and more. Physicians were being hired to address these subspecialty needs and give patients the best care possible.

While audiology was added to the clinic in 1978, with Bruce Vircks as the company's first doctor of audiology, under the branding of Wolfe Audiology, two new products were introduced in the early 1990s: the implantable hearing aid (1992) and resound hearing aid technology (1993).

Innovation exploded in the 1990s as more brilliant ophthalmologists came aboard. Graether, one of the senior-most physicians at the time, created one of his signature surgical tools, the Graether Pupil Expander, in 1996. The tool helps surgeons create a larger pupil without iris damage to make cataract surgery safer. In 1999, Wolfe Eye Clinic was the first in Iowa to perform the intracorneal rings procedure to correct nearsightedness. And in the next decade, Wolfe Eye Clinic surgeons were the first in Iowa to implant FDA-approved multifocal intraocular lenses in 2003 and toric intraocular lenses to correct astigmatism in 2005.

> **But with more technology and improved procedures came the need for more expertise in specific subspecialized fields like cornea, glaucoma, cataract and refractive, pediatrics and strabismus, retina and oculoplastics facial surgery.**

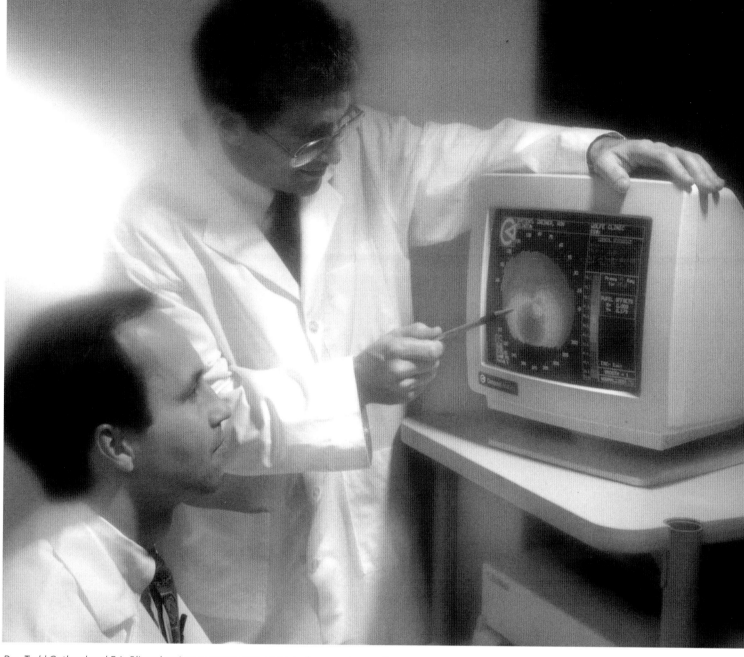

Drs. Todd Gothard and Eric Bligard review a cornea scan on an early computer monitor.

These were just a few of the notable advancements in the decade. With the clinic's influence rising throughout Iowa, quality of care increased with it.

"Every time we have gone into a community, we've raised the quality of care in the community," Graether said. "Because if the existing physicians were going to compete with us, they had to bring up the standard of care somewhere close to ours. I think we've had a profound impact on ophthalmology to the benefit of Iowans."

At the turn of the century, Wolfe Eye Clinic had changed the lives of countless numbers of people. Physicians had performed hundreds of thousands of procedures. The previous two decades were a whirlwind, to be sure. But it was an exciting experience for physicians and team members alike.

In 2000, Wolfe Eye Clinic was now one of the largest eye-care providers in Iowa. With six physical locations and many other outreach centers, the clinic reached almost every part of the state. And the Des Moines location was well on its way to becoming the largest eye-care practice in central Iowa.

"It was such an exhilarating experience," Davison said. "Every two years we opened another office. But when you're young, like I was, you are kind of expecting to do that. Now that I look back, you really appreciate how historically different Wolfe Eye Clinic was from other places. We became a big fish in the small pond of the state of Iowa."

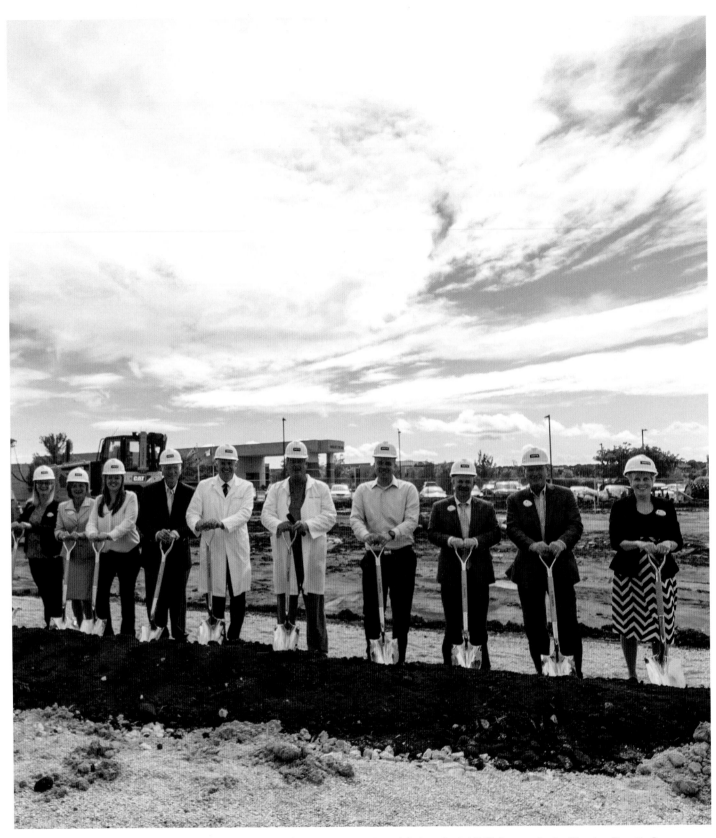

The Wolfe Eye Clinic team at the groundbreaking for the Wolfe Surgery Center. From left: Sara Kraft, Wolfe Surgery Center Director; Danette Pease, Director of Office Operations; Kassandra Trenary, Director of Marketing; Dr. John Graether; Dr. Steven Johnson; Dr. James Davison; Dr. Derek Bitner; Luke Bland, Chief Financial Officer; Kevin Swartz, Chief Executive Officer; Susan Holm, Senior Director of Clinical Services.

STEEPED IN SUCCESS

Wolfe Eye Clinic celebrated 100 years of excellence in 2019. It was a time to honor past innovation, the Wolfe family and high-quality care, but also an opportunity to look forward to the next 100 years.

In the time since 2000, the clinic has seen tremendous growth. New locations, including ones in Waterloo, Iowa City and Ottumwa, expanded the business' reach. More new medical advancements, like the small-incision, no-stitch vitrectomy procedure or improved intraocular lenses, led to better care for patients. Wolfe Eye Clinic has also become more involved with scientific medical and surgical study trials, which give patients opportunities for the newest treatments while also advancing the industry as a whole.

Nine Wolfe Family Vision Centers, staffed with their own full-time optometrists, are located throughout Iowa's rural areas. They provide eye care to mostly underserved communities.

Perhaps one of the biggest and most exciting changes has been the addition of a state-of-the-art, 25,000-square-foot Surgery Center in West Des Moines, which opened in 2019. The Surgery Center provides significantly more space for physicians and is outfitted with the latest and greatest technology. The center has six operating rooms compared to three before in the one built in 2007 in the clinic building, and it has a state-of-the-art Refractive Surgery LASIK Suite and an Oculofacial Plastic Surgery Center. The building also houses the NGENUITY Visualization System for retina surgery.

This new facility is the largest ophthalmologic-specific ambulatory surgery center in the state of Iowa and it has a state-of-the-art Refractive Surgery LASIK Suite and an Oculofacial Plastic Surgery Center.

"It's an astounding facility," Swartz said. "There's really nothing like it in this part of the Midwest."

Davison added: "It's a dream come true. It's huge, and it's really one of the most beautiful centers you will find in the country. I've never seen anything as scientifically luxurious as this. I'm thrilled every time I walk in there."

New subspecialties have emerged in ophthalmology at Wolfe Eye Clinic, including pediatrics (2000) and cosmetic oculoplastics (2019). While oculoplastic in a medical sense has been part of Wolfe Eye Clinic for many years, in 2019, with the addition of a second oculofacial plastic surgeon, Dr. Audrey Ko, Wolfe Eye Clinic focuses more on helping patients with both the functional and cosmetic surgery of the structures around the eye. This may include injectables such as Botox, or surgery near the eyelids, the eyebrows, the lacrimal tear system and the tissues of the orbit area surrounding the eye.

100 ACTS OF KINDNESS

To commemorate the 100-year anniversary, Wolfe Eye Clinic wanted to give back to the communities that meant so much to it over the last century. That's how the 100 Acts of Kindness initiative was born. In 2019, Wolfe Eye Clinic gave back to communities by volunteering and donating time and money. Examples include sponsoring Marshalltown's Oktemberfest celebration, helping build Habitat for Humanity houses or donating physician time to performing crucial eye procedures on underprivileged individuals around the state and in underprivileged countries.

"It meant so much for us to give back," Swartz said. "We wanted to find anything that we could do to help, and our experience really ran the gamut. I think that was pretty cool. Any organization can donate money and feel good about it — and rightfully so — but we really wanted our people to get involved in the community."

Making it to 100 years in business is a hard task, but it's particularly difficult in the medical industry, where quality of care is paramount. Now with more than 45 physicians and 40 locations across Iowa, Wolfe Eye Clinic continues to be on the cutting edge, always looking to improve patient experiences.

That's what has distinguished the clinic from the rest of the industry for the past 100 years, and it's what will continue to propel the business into its next century of operation.

"The only way you can make it to 100 years of success is by being fair, honest and by treating people well," Davison said. "This is a service business, and we try to take care of people as best we can, and they know it. We love our patients, and I think they know that too. That's how we got to 100 years — by taking good care of and loving the patients and families we serve."

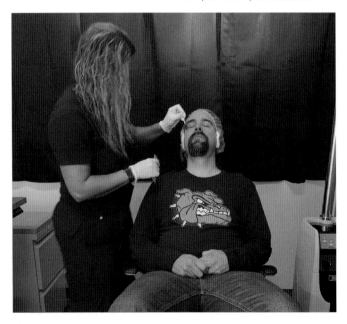

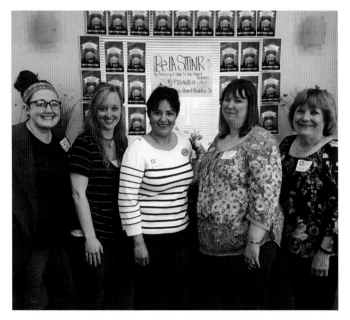

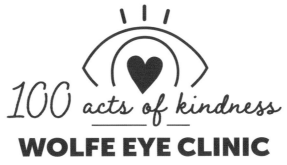

WOLFE EYE CLINIC

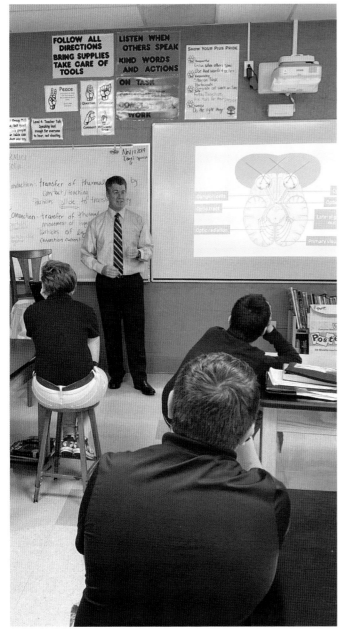

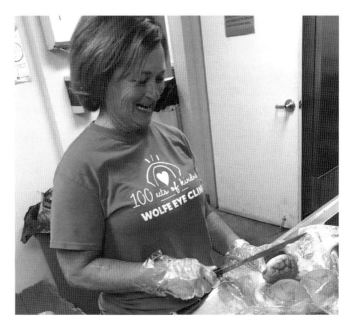

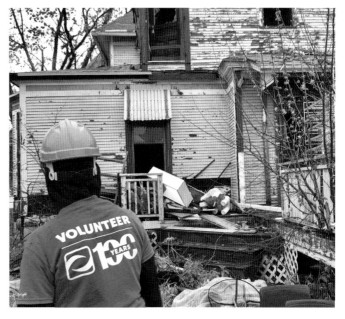

For Wolfe Eye Clinic's 100-year anniversary, doctors and team members performed 100 Acts of Kindness in various communities, including volunteering, donations and more.

An early pamphlet showcasing options and prices for bifocal lenses, which are used with eyeglasses.

THROUGHOUT THE YEARS

1919

Dr. Otis R. Wolfe travels to Marshalltown to open new clinic in partnership with eyes, nose and throat specialist Dr. Frederick L. Wahrer.

1925

Dr. Otis R. Wolfe and Dr. Frederick L. Wahrer perform and publish the results of their first intracapsular cataract surgeries (The Barraquer Method) in the United States.

The agreement for Dr. Otis Rudolph Wolfe to start Wolfe Eye Clinic in the Masonic Temple in downtown Marshalltown.

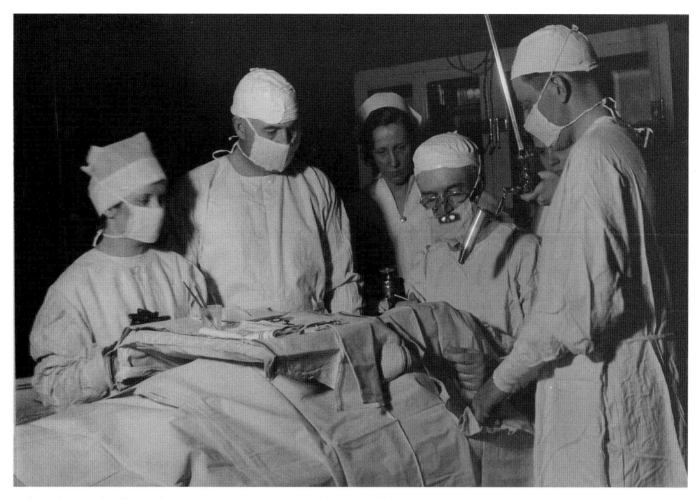

In the early years of Wolfe Eye Clinic, cataracts surgeries made up the majority of procedures. In this photo, doctors and nurses assist Dr. Russell Watt on one such surgery.

1927

Dr. Otis R. Wolfe travels to Spain to further study the Barraquer method.

1931

Cataract suction-aspiration surgery performed on children by Dr. Otis R. Wolfe, who continues to improve the procedure throughout the next decade.

1936

Wolfe Foundation established.

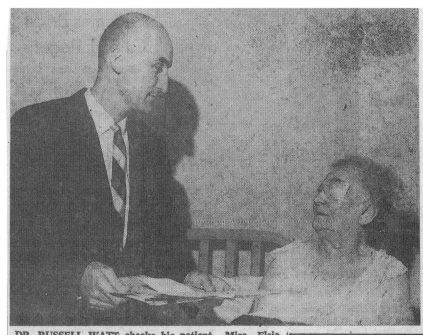

DR. RUSSELL WATT checks his patient, Miss Elsie Bartling, on whom he performed the first corneal transplant ever to be done in Marshalltown. (T-R Staff Photo)

Eye Transplant Operation Performed in City Hospital

after death, but they may fail to notify their relatives of the intention and then are buried without the donation being made.

Explaining how the eye bank operates, Dr. Watt said that immediately after the

1940-46

Dr. Otis R Wolfe's three sons join the practice after serving in World War II. Dr. Otis D. Wolfe and Dr. Russell Wolfe were ophthalmologists; Dr. Henry Wolfe an optometrist.

1959

First board-certified ophthalmologist joins Wolfe Eye Clinic.

1960

Wolfe Eye Clinic is the first provider outside of a university setting to perform corneal transplantation.

1960-65

Introduction of several surgical techniques to Wolfe Eye Clinic to treat retinal disease including the scleral buckle and in 1965, Xenon Arc photocoagulation of the retina. These procedures had formerly been the exclusive province of a university setting.

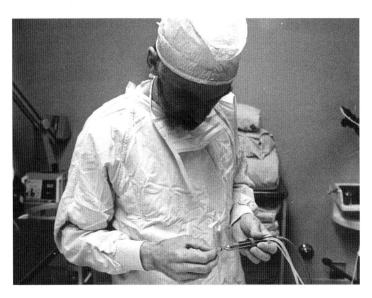

Dr. Russell Watt examines a phacoemulsifier, a utensil used during cataracts surgeries that Wolfe Eye Clinic was one of the first to adopt.

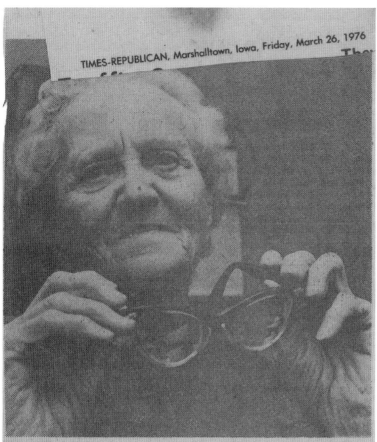

TIMES-REPUBLICAN, Marshalltown, Iowa, Friday, March 26, 1976

PERFECT VISION has been restored to Miss **Clara Breniman** (pictured), age 100, of Grinnell. She underwent a sees as well as anyone. A former seamstress, she says she will now do some sewing in her spare time. She

Clara Brenlman underwent eye surgery at Wolfe Eye Clinic, restoring her vision, she told the Marshalltown Times-Republican in 1976. During the 1960s and '70s, thousands of patient lives were changed thanks to Wolfe Eye Clinic procedures.

1966

Cataract surgery first accomplished using an operating microscope

1969

Wolfe Foundation Lecture, an endowed lecture series for ophthalmologists across the Midwest, is founded. Hosted at the University of Iowa College of Medicine's Department of Ophthalmology and Visual Sciences, Wolfe Foundation Lecture is held annually to this day.

1972

First small-incision phacoemulsification surgery for cataracts performed in Iowa at Wolfe Eye Clinic.

1975

First artificial intraocular lens (IOL) implanted as a replacement lens during cataract surgery.

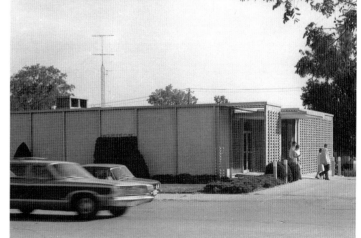

An outside shot of the Marshalltown office, which was built in 1961.

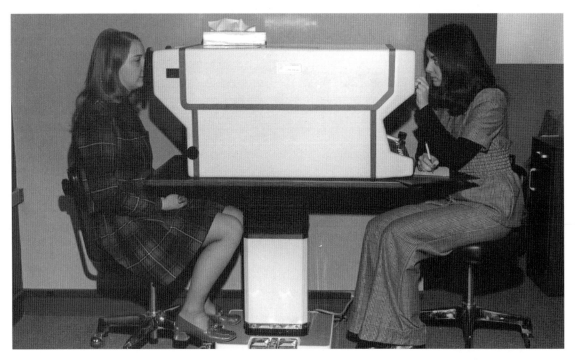

Specialty trained technicians have been key to the utilization of new vision testing technologies over the years at Wolfe Eye Clinic.

1977

Wolfe Eye Clinic begins offering facial plastic surgery as well as ears, nose and throat (ENT) care and treatment services, hiring first otolaryngologist on staff.

1978

Retina laser surgery first performed at Wolfe Eye Clinic using water cooled Argon laser.

1981

Dr. James Davison begins training optometrists across the state of Iowa.

1981

Wolfe Eye Clinic performs first pars plana vitrectomy (PPV) to help treat a variety of retinal diseases including macular holes and retinal detachments.

A Wolfe Eye Clinic optometrist evaluates a patient's eyesight.

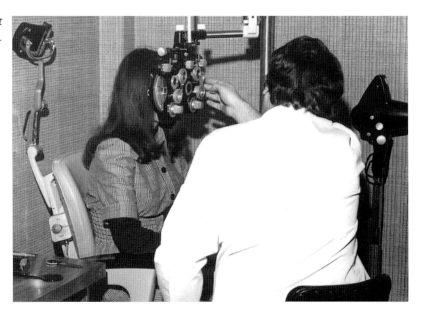

1983

Wolfe Audiology is founded, offering patients comprehensive hearing loss evaluation and treatment services.

1984

Refractive surgery is first performed at Wolfe Eye Clinic to reduce reliance on eyeglasses or contact lenses.

Doctor: Ray 'doing well' after surgery

Gov. Robert Ray is expected to return to Des Moines today after successful surgery in Marshalltown Friday to correct a cataract problem in his right eye.

Dr. John Graether, an ophthalmic surgeon who performed the operation, said Ray was "doing very well" and should be able to resume most of his normal activities within two weeks.

Graether said Ray spent about 35 minutes in surgery before he returned to his room at Marshalltown Area Community Hospital about 10:30 a.m. Friday.

In simple terms, a cataract is a clouding of the lens of the eye. The lens, which is behind the cornea or "clear window" at the front of the eye, focuses images on the retina.

Graether explained that he had removed all but the covering of the lens of Ray's right eye and replaced it with a plastic lens called an "intraocular implant."

Common Operation

Cataract surgery is one of the most common operations in the country, Graether said. The Wolfe eye clinic in Marshalltown has performed about 4,000 lens implants since 1975, and about 95 percent of them resulted in improved vision.

Graether said the governor had been sedated and given a local anesthetic before the operation, which was done with the aid of an operating microscope.

He said he does not expect any complications that would require further eye surgery, but he said Ray won't be fully recovered for six weeks to two months and will have to refrain from strenuous exercise or lifting.

Checkups Scheduled

Ray will return to Marshalltown in two weeks and again in a month for checkups, the second to determine whether he needs a different prescription for his glasses, which he wears primarily for reading.

Graether said Ray was in good spirits after the surgery, but slightly groggy.

"He said he liked the sedation very much," Graether said. "He said it's the best rest he's had in some time."

An article in the Des Moines Register detailing Dr. John Graether's procedure on Gov. Robert Ray.

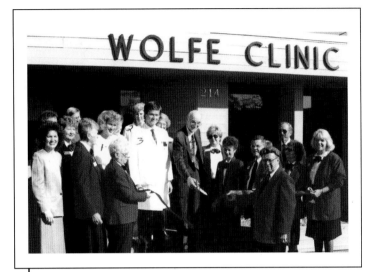

1984

Wolfe Eye Clinic first expands, opening a second main location in West Des Moines, Iowa.

1985

Wolfe Eye Clinic cataract specialist, Dr. John Graether, co-develops capsulorhexis technique for cataract surgery, the standard technique used throughout the world.

A newspaper article detailing Dr. Otis D. Wolfe's retirement in the 1990s. The retirement marked the first time a Wolfe family member wasn't practicing at Wolfe Eye Clinic in 73 years.

LOOKING AT RETIREMENT

Wolfe says goodbye to eye clinic

By GENE RAFFENSPERGER
REGISTER STAFF WRITER

When the new year dawns in Marshalltown Wednesday, it will mark the first year in 73 that a Wolfe has not been in medical practice there, specializing in treating eyes.

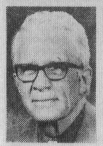

Wolfe
Nearly 80

Dr. Otis D. Wolfe, the last of three brothers who with their father established the prestigious Wolfe Clinic here, has retired.

"I'll be 80 in January. It was just time," Wolfe said from his Marshalltown home Friday. "I want to pursue other things now."

Those other things likely will be travel, photography and gardening, to name just three of his interests.

Wolfe Clinic will continue under that name. It now has a staff of about 160, including people at satellite clinics in West Des Moines, Cedar Falls, Cedar Rapids and Carroll.

Wolfe said the clinic had its beginnings in 1946, but traces its roots to 1918.

That was the year when his father, the late Dr. Otis R. Wolfe, started his medical practice in Marshalltown, specializing in treating eyes, ears and noses.

Wolfe had four sons, three of whom eventually entered the practice with their father after World War II in what was the beginning of the Wolfe Clinic.

The sons are Dr. Russell Wolfe, an ophthalmologist, now retired in Arkansas; Dr. Henry Wolfe, an optometrist, now retired in Texas; and Dr. Otis D. Wolfe, an ophthalmologist, who will remain in Marshalltown.

Wolfe was asked why the clinic kept its headquarters in Marshalltown. "We had an unusual arrangement, started by my father, with the hospital in Marshalltown. We had our own department there, our own surgery and even our own nurses. I think this created a neighborly atmosphere among our staff and our patients."

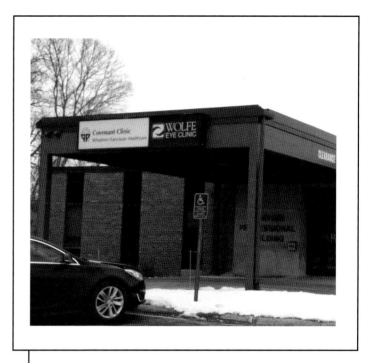

GROWTH THROUGHOUT IOWA

1986

Wolfe Eye Clinic opens a third main location in Fort Dodge, Iowa.

1987

Wolfe Eye Clinic opens a fourth main location in Cedar Falls, Iowa.

1988

Wolfe Eye Clinic cataract specialist, Dr. Russell Watt, first in Iowa to implant a foldable intraocular lens (IOL) as an artificial lens replacement during cataract surgery.

Wolfe Eye Clinic opens in F.D.

By MIKE HEFFERN
Messenger staff writer

The Fort Dodge branch office of the Wolfe Eye Clinic officially opened for business in the Fort Dodge Medical Center Monday.

The office will see approximately 30 patients a day from all over northwest Iowa, according to Jeanette Johnson, in charge of the receptionist staff in the remodeled, 4,000-square-foot wing on the ground floor of the Medical Center.

THE FIRST SURGERY, an intraocular lens implant, will be performed this morning, said Dr. John Graether, one of six rotating ophthalmologists who will be seeing patients at the Fort Dodge office.

The Wolfe Eye Clinic is based in Marshalltown and has another branch office in West Des Moines. In 1985, the clinic treated 60,000 patients at the two locations.

"We will continue to rotate until a resident ophthalmologist is hired," Graether said.

"We are primarily a referral practice, except for those who have very specific eye disease problems," Graether said. "We are not equipped for routine examinations."

THE NEW FACILITY will employ an operation staff of seven, including four local employees. Johnson said the staff will be seeing "30 patients a day to start with and more later, depending on when we get a full-time ophthalmologist."

Graether said they are still trying to recruit the resident ophthalmologist.

Graether and the new staff were welcomed to the new location by the ambassadors of the Greater Fort Dodge Area Chamber of Commerce in a ribbon cutting ceremony Monday afternoon.

More than $50,000 was expended to remodel the wing. The figure does not include the cost of equipment, which was either purchased new or transferred from Marshalltown.

THE WOLFE EYE Clinic was founded in 1919 by Dr. Otis Wolfe, whose son, Dr. Otis D. Wolfe, is one of the seven ophthalmologists at the Marshalltown clinic.

The new ophthalmic clinic brings to 10 the number of specialties found in the Medical Center.

The pediatrics offices, which formerly occupied the Wolfe Clinic space, have moved to the upper level.

Other specialties found in the Medical Center are family practice, surgery, obstetrics and gynecology, radiology, orthopedic surgery, dermatology, internal medicine and otorhinolaryngology (ear, nose and throat).

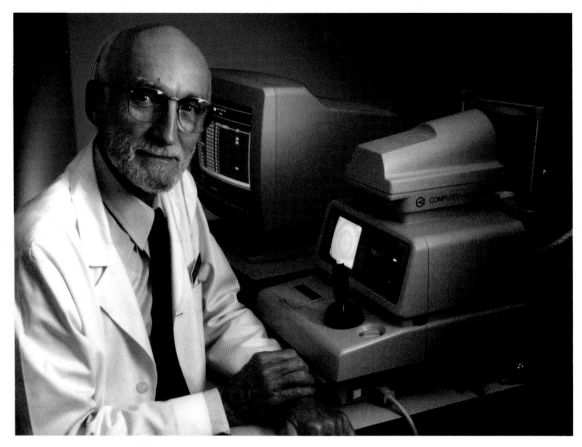

Dr. Russell Watt was one of the early innovators at Wolfe Eye Clinic, which performed many firsts in the 1970s, '80s and '90s.

1991

Wolfe Eye Clinic cataract specialists introduce one-stitch or no-stitch cataract surgery to Iowa and are some of the first surgeons in the world to use this technology.

1991

Wolfe Eye Clinic otolaryngologist surgeon, Dr. Michael Hill, first in Iowa to use Candela laser to remove birthmarks such as port wine stains and other vascular abnormalities of the skin.

1991

Wolfe Eye Clinic opens a fifth main location in Cedar Rapids, Iowa.

1992

Wolfe Eye Clinic cataract and retina surgeon, Dr. Norman Woodlief, performs basic research on capsular opacification reduction.

I. Marshalltown, Iowa, October 23, 1993

Raymond Swift returns to MMSC and repeats eye surgery history

By NORMA LYNCH
T-R Staff Writer

History repeated itself in Marshalltown Thursday when a Central Iowa man who had been the subject of a revolutionary medical procedure 21 years ago came back to do it again.

Raymond Swift, a 79-year-old Gilman farmer, was the first person in the Midwest to receive small-incision cataract surgery in December 1972.

"It was revolutionary at that time," says Dr. John Graether, M.D., a physician with Marshalltown's Wolfe Eye Clinic, who performed the pioneering 1972 surgery on Swift's right eye.

The Gilman farmer returned to Marshalltown Medical & Surgical Center this week and had the same procedure performed on his left eye.

The circumstances were strikingly similar — same hospital, same doctor, even the same scrub nurse, Janice Faber.

"It's much easier now," was Swift's assessment of the 1993 procedure compared to the surgery in 1972.

Following Thursday's surgery, the doctors and nurses held a small ceremony in Swift's hospital room, where Graether presented the patient with a cake marking the special occasion.

The procedure that made Swift a Midwest celebrity in the field of eye surgery is called phacoemulsification. Before the introduction of that technique, cataract surgery had depended on wide incisions. The new small-incision technique, which was pioneered in the Midwest in a Marshalltown hospital operating room, has now become so common that around 1,500 a year are performed annually at MMSC.

When Smith was operated on in 1972, he was admitted to the hospital and had a one- to two-day recuperation stay.

On Thursday, he was admitted as an outpatient and left the hospital about an hour and a half after his surgery. He returned for a quick checkup the following day and the technique was complete.

"He did very well with both surgeries," Graether said afterwards.

The doctor joked with Swift Thursday following the surgery, telling him the phacoemulsification technique had been thoroughly tested before it was completed on him in 1972. "You followed a large series of cats," he said, laughing.

The patient's wife, Enza Swift, says although 21 years have passed, the surgery and procedures for her husband all seem very familiar. "Not that much has changed," she said.

One change which has improved vision for those receiving the small-incision surgery is today's standard practice of inserting an implant during the surgery. In Swift's first operation, implants were not used, and it wasn't until several years later he received an implant in his right eye.

The cataract surgery became a one-day procedure in 1984, according to John Cahill, public relations director for the hospital.

He says outpatient surgeries have become commonplace in several health areas. "You are going to continue to see more and more outpatient procedures," he said.

He attributes the increases to a combination of changes in the health industry including medical advances, the need for cost efficiencies, and a recognition by medical experts that patients recover better at home.

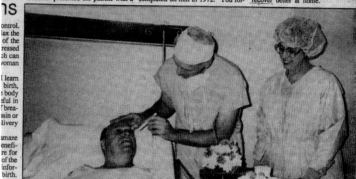

A newspaper article showcasing Wolfe Eye Clinic's superb eye history experience and success on a patient.them in-house to work hand-in-hand.

1992

First use of an implantable hearing aid device, the Xomed implant, by Wolfe Eye Clinic Audiologist, Dr. Bruce Vircks.

1992

First use of "eye drop" topical anesthesia for cataract surgery to increase patient comfort and reduce risk during cataract surgery.

1993

Wolfe Eye Clinic changes to sutureless temporal clear cornea incisions for cataract surgery

1993

Wolfe Audiology first uses refined digital hearing aid technology to better address each patient's specific hearing needs.

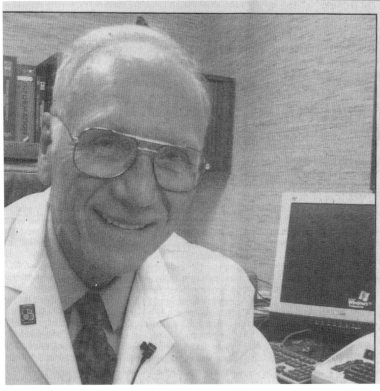

Local physician credited with a medical invention

By RYAN BRINKS
T-R Staff Writer

A decade-old medical invention by a local Wolfe Eye Clinic specialist may finally take off now that circumstances have turned the industry's attention back to it.

What may become the defining contribution of the 43-year career of Marshalltown's own John Graether, M.D. is his pupil expander device used during cataract surgery.

Just now slowing down at the age of 75, Graether is very much part of the model that has helped make Wolfe Eye Clinic as respected as it is today.

In correcting urination problems, Tamsulosin, or Flomax, also paralyzes dilator muscles in the normally firm iris of the eye, making it floppy.

"The pupil expander proved to be a very good solution to the problem," Graether said.

The need for the pupil expander made itself apparent to Graether after he struggled through a cataract operation in a patient with a small pupil sometime in the late 1980s and set his mind to searching for a solution.

"Devising the pupil expander was easy. The problem was finding a way to get

1994

Wolfe Eye Clinic refractive specialists first perform automated lamellar keratoplasty to correct high degree nearsightedness (myopia).

1994

Wolfe Eye Clinic participated in FDA trials for laser vision correction with the excimer laser (Dr. Steven C. Johnson and Dr. Todd A. Gothard).

1995

The Clinic implants the first foldable acrylic intraocular lens in Iowa

1996

Wolfe Eye Clinic LASIK specialists, Dr. Todd Gothard and Dr. Steven Johnson, first in Iowa to perform LASIK laser eye surgery with the excimer laser.

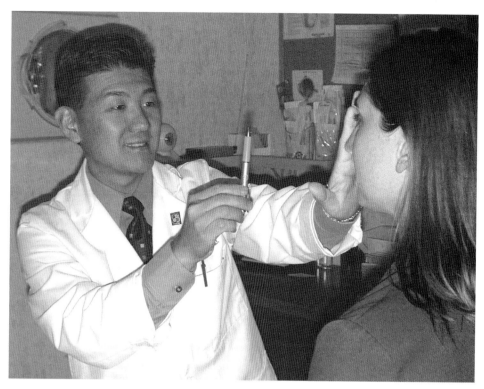

Dr. Donny Suh was the first pediatric ophthalmologist at Wolfe Eye Clinic.

1996

Wolfe Eye Clinic cataract specialist, Dr. John Graether, invents the Graether Pupil Expander to mechanically dilate the eye's pupil and maintain dilation during cataract surgery and artificial intraocular lens (IOL) implantation. The device is adopted by surgeons across the globe.

1996

Wolfe Family Vision Center is developed to provide integrated primary family eye care, with the first Wolfe Family Vision Center opening in Fairfield, Iowa.

1997

Wolfe Eye Clinic merges with Iowa Eye Care Physicians, P.C. and opens a sixth main location in Ames, Iowa.

1998

Wolfe Family Vision Center opens a second location in Webster City, Iowa, followed by a third location in Waverly, Iowa.

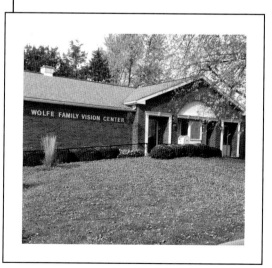

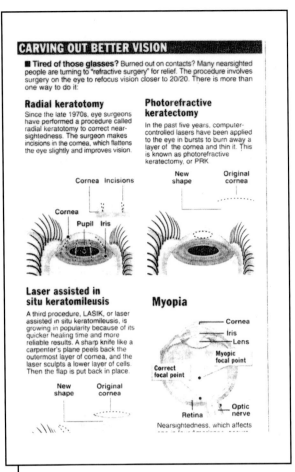

CARVING OUT BETTER VISION

■ **Tired of those glasses?** Burned out on contacts? Many nearsighted people are turning to "refractive surgery" for relief. The procedure involves surgery on the eye to refocus vision closer to 20/20. There is more than one way to do it:

Radial keratotomy

Since the late 1970s, eye surgeons have performed a procedure called radial keratotomy to correct nearsightedness. The surgeon makes incisions in the cornea, which flattens the eye slightly and improves vision.

Photorefractive keratectomy

In the past five years, computer-controlled lasers have been applied to the eye in bursts to burn away a layer of the cornea and thin it. This is known as photorefractive keratectomy, or PRK.

Laser assisted in situ keratomileusis

A third procedure, LASIK, or laser assisted in situ keratomileusis, is growing in popularity because of its quicker healing time and more reliable results. A sharp knife like a carpenter's plane peels back the outermost layer of cornea, and the laser sculpts a lower layer of cells. Then the flap is put back in place.

Myopia

Nearsightedness, which affects

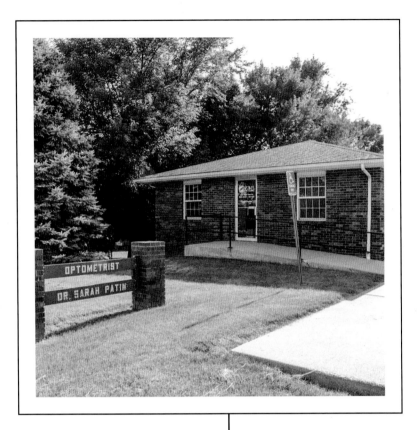

1999

More than 80,000 small-incision cataract operations have been performed at the Wolfe Eye Clinic in its history. More than 9,000 refractive surgeries have been performed to correct nearsightedness, farsightedness and astigmatism.

1999

Wolfe Eye Clinic refractive specialists, Dr. Steven Johnson and Dr. Todd Gothard, first in central and eastern Iowa to perform intracorneal ring segment, also known as Intacs, to correct nearsightedness (myopia).

1999

Wolfe Eye Clinic retina specialists begin using transpupillary thermotherapy (TTT) to treat specific forms of age-related macular degeneration (AMD).

1999

Wolfe Family Vision Center opens two more locations in Toledo and Traer, Iowa.

A NEW CENTURY BEGINS

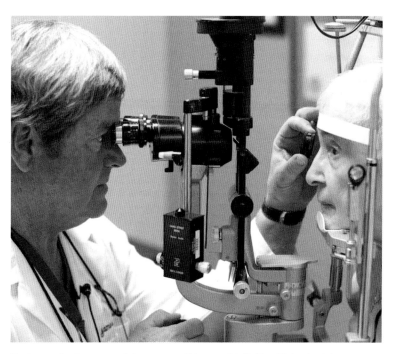

Dr. James Davison, one of the most well-known Wolfe Eye Clinic physicians, performs an evaluation of a patient.

2000

Wolfe Eye Clinic opens a seventh main location in Waterloo, Iowa.

2000

10,000 LASIK procedures and 100,000 cataract procedures have been performed at Wolfe Eye Clinic.

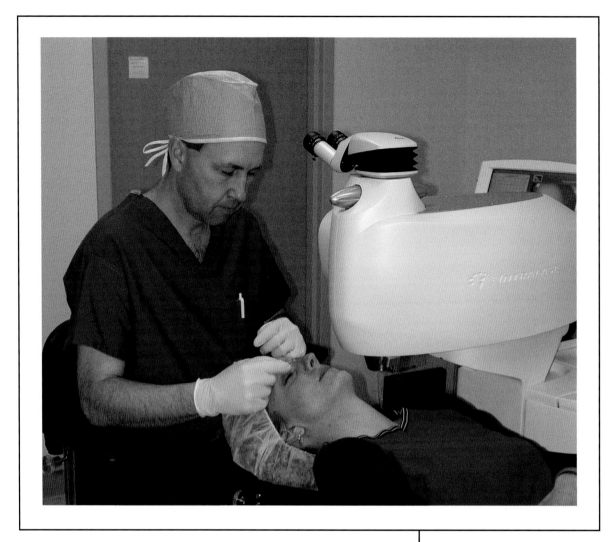

2000

Wolfe Eye Clinic retina specialists begin using photodynamic therapy (PDT) to treat specific forms of age-related macular degeneration (AMD).

2001

First use of feeder vessel treatment with high-speed indocyanine green (ICG) angiography at Wolfe Eye Clinic to treat specific forms of age-related macular degeneration (AMD).

2002

Wolfe Eye Clinic retina specialist, Dr. David Saggau, first in Iowa to perform small-incision, no-stitch vitrectomy surgery to treat retina disease. This advanced procedure minimizes trauma to the eye and is more comfortable for the patient.

2002

Wolfe Eye Clinic LASIK specialists first in Iowa to obtain and use IntraLASE™ Femtosecond Laser to create corneal flaps for laser vision correction. Adoption of this laser made Wolfe Eye Clinic the first in the state to offer patients 100% all-laser, bladeless LASIK, that medical standard for LASIK surgery to-date.

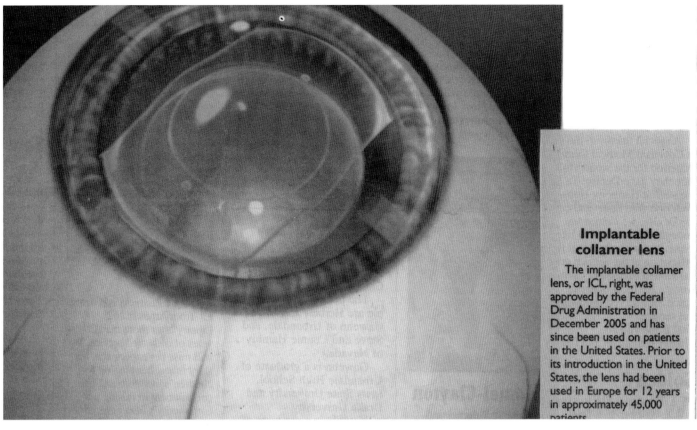

The implantable collamer lens, implemented in the 2000s, was a much-improved replacement during cataract surgery.

2002

Wolfe Eye Clinic cataract surgeon, Dr. Daniel Vos, first in Iowa to perform laser-assisted cataract surgery using the Dodick PhotoLysisTM Surgical System.

2002

Wolfe Family Vision Center opens a sixth location in Sac City, Iowa.

2003

First selective laser trabeculoplasty (SLT) procedure is performed by Wolfe Eye Clinic glaucoma specialist, Dr. John Trible, to lower intraocular pressure and improve the treatment of glaucoma.

2003

Wolfe Eye Clinic cataract surgeon, Dr. James Davison, first in Iowa to implant AcrySof® IQ ReSTOR® multifocal intraocular lens (IOL) as an artificial lens replacement during cataract surgery, helping to eliminate the need for glasses post-cataract surgery.

Wolfe Eye Clinic performs routine eye checkups on patients to ensure the highest quality of care.

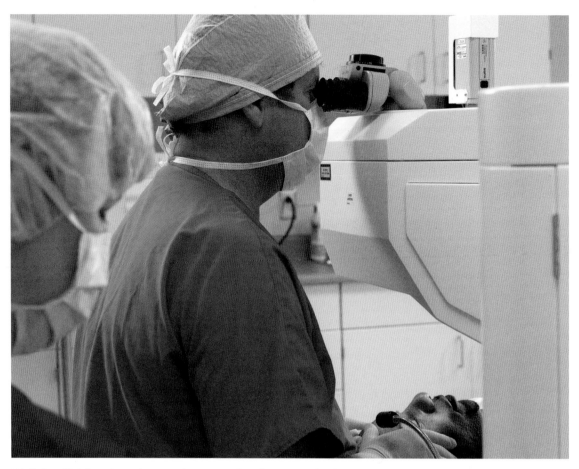

Wolfe Eye Clinic has always been on the cutting edge of surgery technology, giving patients the best care available.

2004

Wolfe Family Vision Center opens a seventh location in Story City, Iowa, and an eighth location in Sigourney, Iowa.

2005

First intravitreal injection for the treatment of wet-type Age-Related Macular Degeneration (AMD).

2006

First in Iowa to implant a toric intraocular Lens (IOL) as an artificial lens replacement that treats for astigmatism during cataract surgery.

Dr. David Saggau, Dr. Donny Suh, Dr. Steven Johnson and Dr. James Davison break ground on the new West Des Moines Clinic, which opened in 2004.

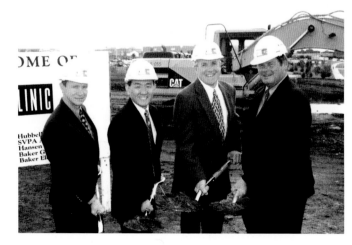

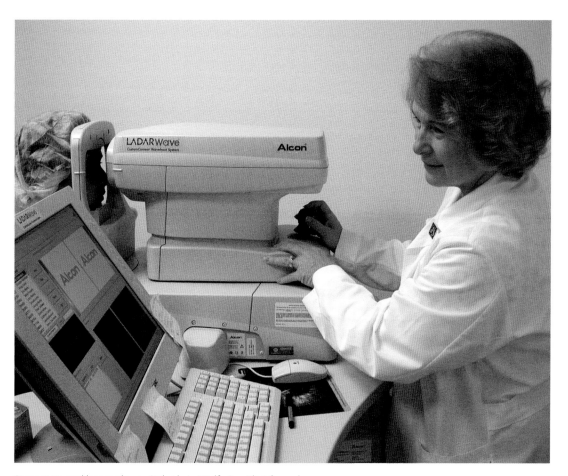

Computers and lasers play a vital role in Wolfe Eye Clinic's work.

2006

Wolfe Eye Clinic surgeon, Dr. Daniel Vos, was the first in Iowa to place an Implantable Contact Lens (ICL), as an alternative refractive treatment for patients who did not qualify for LASIK vision correction surgery.

2007

Wolfe Surgery Center opens with three operating rooms inside of the West Des Moines Wolfe Eye Clinic building. At this time, more than 150,000 small-incision cataract surgeries and over 25,000 laser vision correction procedures have been performed at Wolfe Eye Clinic.

2007

First in Iowa to obtain and begin using Allegretto Wave® Eye-Q Excimer Laser as a vision correction laser for LASIK laser eye surgery.

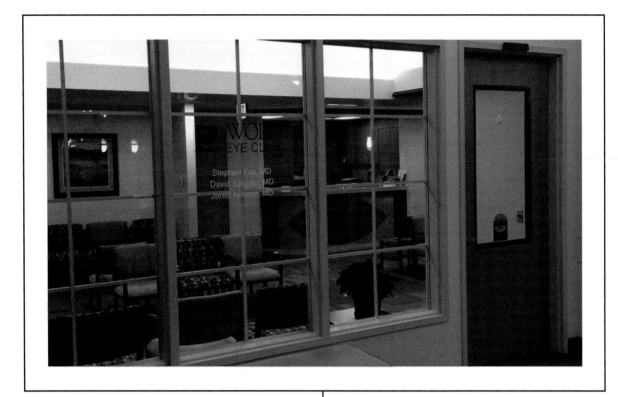

2007

Wolfe Eye Clinic first in Iowa to begin performing glaucoma surgery with the use of a Trabectome (Dr. John R. Trible).

2009

More than 31,000 refractive surgeries have been performed to correct nearsightedness, farsightedness and astigmatism.

2011

Wolfe Eye Clinic opens an eighth main location In Spencer, Iowa.

2011

First in Iowa to obtain and begin using the advanced WaveLight® FS200 Laser, continuing Wolfe Eye Clinic's history of using bladeless technology to create corneal flaps for vision correction during LASIK laser eye surgery.

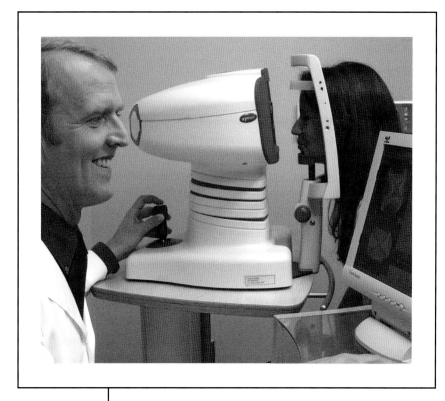

2012

Wolfe Eye Clinic First in Iowa to obtain and begin using Alcon LenSx® Laser System used in conjunction with laser-assisted cataract surgery.

2012

More than 165,000 small-incision cataract surgeries have been performed at Wolfe Eye Clinic and over 37,000 refractive surgeries have been performed to correct nearsightedness, farsightedness and astigmatism.

2013

Wolfe Eye Clinic is pronounced number one site for Pediatric Eye Disease Investigator Group (PEDIG), a national collaborative network dedicated to clinical research in childhood eye disorders such as strabismus and amblyopia.

2013

Wolfe Eye Clinic opens a ninth main location in Iowa City, Iowa.

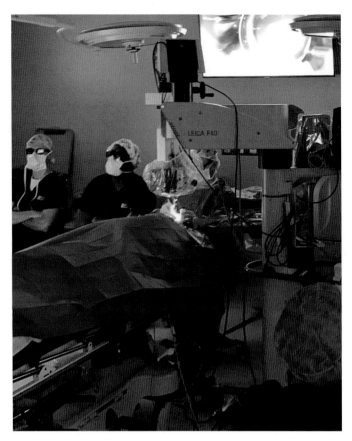

Advanced vitreoretinal surgeries can be performed with surgeons and staff wearing polarized glasses to provide highly detailed 3D depth perception while viewing a 55 inch computer monitor.

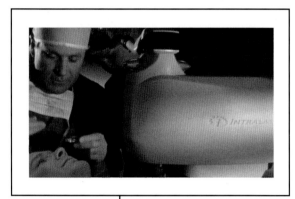

2014

Wolfe Eye Clinic merges with Heartland Eye Care and opens a tenth Wolfe Eye Clinic main location Ottumwa, Iowa and ninth Wolfe Family Vision Center in Albia, Iowa.

2014

More than 40,000 LASIK laser vision correction procedures and over 175,000 cataract procedures have been performed at Wolfe Eye Clinic.

2015

Wolfe Eye Clinic first in Iowa to obtain and begin using WaveLight® EX500 Excimer Laser as a vision correction laser for LASIK laser eye surgery.

2017

First in Iowa and one of 32 practices nationally to use Alcon NGENUITY® 3D Visualization System to enhance the performance of vitreoretinal surgery.

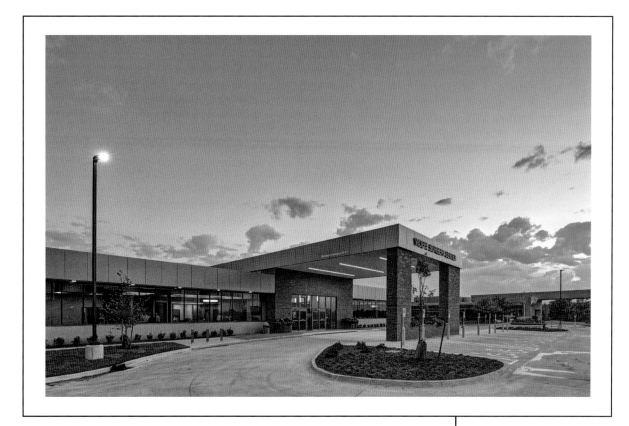

2017

Vitreoretinal Disease and Surgery Fellowship is founded at Wolfe Eye Clinic.

2018

Wolfe Eye Clinic opens an 11th main location in Pleasant Hill, Iowa.

2019

Wolfe Eye Clinic celebrates its 100-year anniversary.

2019

Wolfe Surgery Center opens in West Des Moines as the largest ophthalmology surgery center in the Midwest.

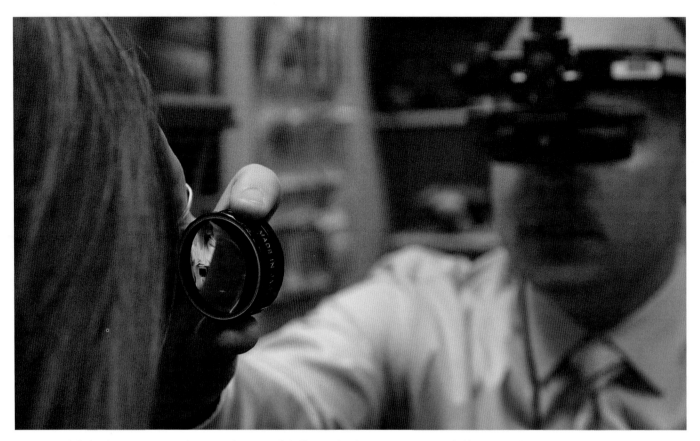

Pediatric ophthalmology continues to become a big part of Wolfe Eye Clinic's care, most recently led by Dr. Derek Bitner.

2019

Wolfe Eye Clinic cornea specialist, Dr. Matthew Rauen, implants first toric implantable contact lens (ICL) in Iowa, expanding vision correction options for patients with astigmatism who do not qualify for LASIK laser eye surgery.

2019

Wolfe Eye Clinic cataract surgeon, Dr. James Davison is first in Iowa to implant Alcon PanOptix® Trifocal Intraocular Lens (IOL) as an artificial lens replacement during cataract surgery, improving vision at multiple distances and reducing the need for glasses post-cataract surgery.

2019

Wolfe Eye Clinic merges with Children's Eye Clinic, a leading pediatric ophthalmology clinic in West Des Moines owned by Dr. Jean Spencer.

2019

First Retina Fellow graduate from Wolfe Eye Clinic fellowship program, Dr. Deepak Mangla.

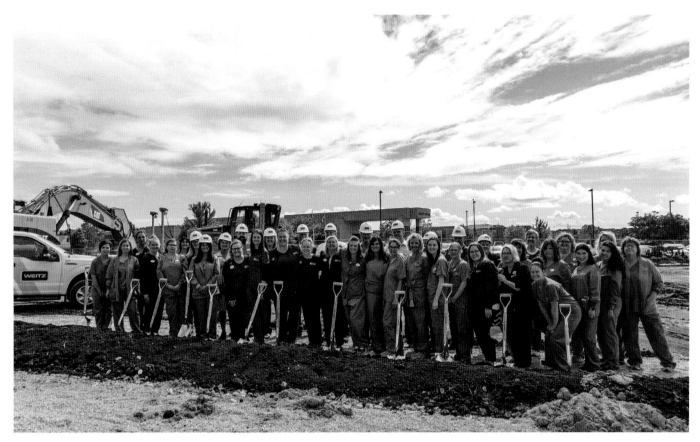

The Wolfe Surgery Center team poses for a photo during groundbreaking of the West Des Moines Surgery Center.

2019

Over 330,000 cataract procedures have been performed at Wolfe Eye Clinic.

2019

More than 340,000 anti-vascular endothelial growth factor (VEGF) intravitreal injections have been administered at Wolfe Eye Clinic.

2019

Over 46,000 LASIK vision correction procedures have been performed at Wolfe Eye Clinic.

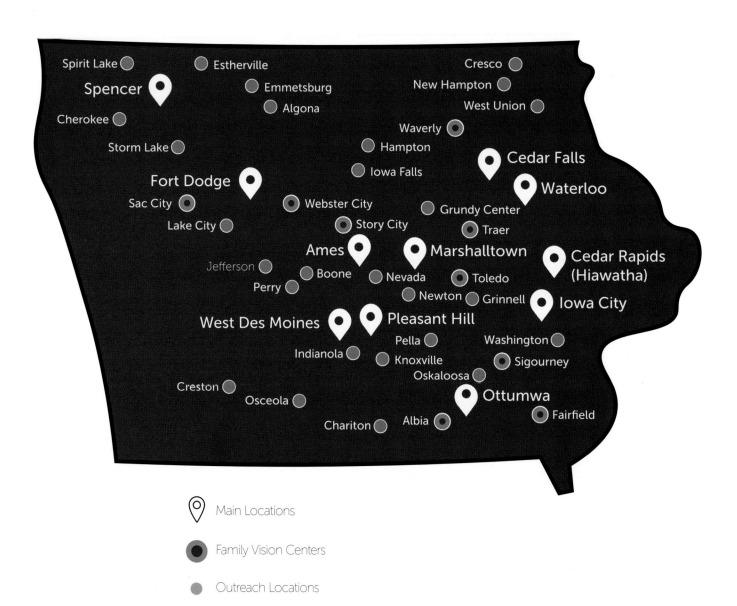

Spirit Lake ⊙   Estherville ⊙   Cresco ⊙
Spencer ◉   New Hampton ⊙
                       Emmetsburg ⊙   West Union ⊙
Cherokee ⊙   Algona ⊙
                                              Waverly ⊙
Storm Lake ⊙   Hampton ⊙
                                              Cedar Falls ◉
Fort Dodge ◉   Iowa Falls ⊙
Sac City ⊙   Waterloo ◉
                       Webster City ⊙   Grundy Center ⊙
Lake City ⊙   Story City ⊙   Traer ⊙
                                                        Cedar Rapids
Ames ◉   Marshalltown ◉   (Hiawatha)
Jefferson ⊙   Nevada ⊙   Toledo ⊙
Perry ⊙   Boone ⊙   Newton ⊙   Grinnell ⊙   Iowa City ◉

West Des Moines ◉ Pleasant Hill ◉
                       Pella ⊙   Washington ⊙
Indianola ⊙   Knoxville ⊙   Sigourney ⊙
Creston ⊙   Oskaloosa ⊙
Osceola ⊙   Ottumwa ◉
              Chariton ⊙   Albia ⊙   Fairfield ⊙

⊚ Main Locations

● Family Vision Centers

● Outreach Locations

LOCATIONS

Across Iowa

LOCATION EXPANSION

Based in Marshalltown for the majority of its history, Wolfe Eye Clinic has expanded to 11 main clinics throughout Iowa. That number almost reaches 50 when including Wolfe Eye Clinic Family Vision Centers, Outreach Offices and the state-of-the-art Surgery Center.

11
Main Locations

9
Family Vision Centers

27
Outreach Offices

MAIN
LOCATIONS

Each main clinic provides its own high level of care,
from cataracts to pediatrics to corneal disease.
Every location has its own story, too. They were all
folded into the Wolfe Eye Clinic family in different
ways, but they all operate with the same patient-
centric approach.

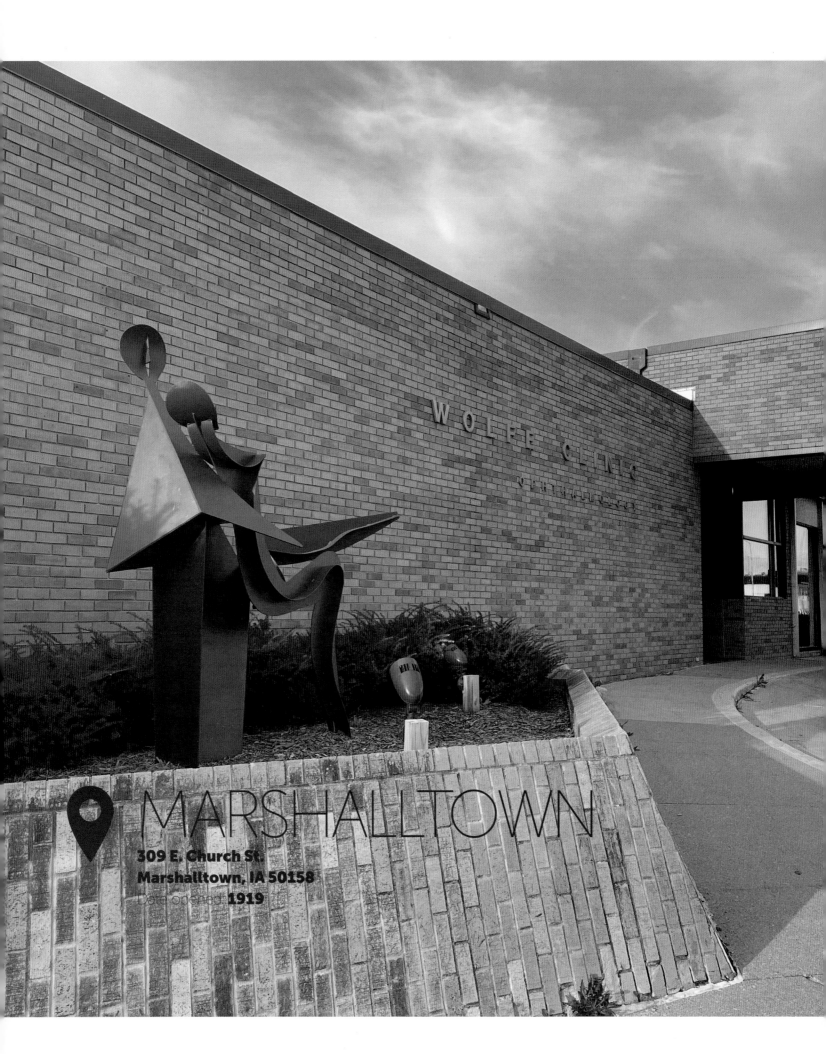

MARSHALLTOWN

309 E. Church St.
Marshalltown, IA 50158
Date opened **1919**

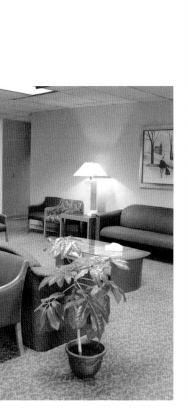

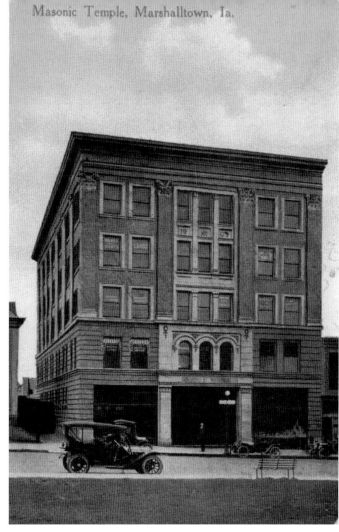

Marshalltown has been the central location for Wolfe Eye Clinic throughout its history. It's where Dr. Otis R. Wolfe, the founder of Wolfe Eye Clinic, decided to start his business back in 1919, on the fourth floor of the Masonic Temple Building (pictured above, right) in downtown Marshalltown. Original services included eyes, ears, nose and throat care.

But Wolfe continued to push the business toward eye care and eventually named it Wolfe Cataract Clinic to reflect the groundbreaking cataract surgeries he performed. Even as early as the 1930s, individuals from around the United States traveled to Marshalltown to undergo procedures at the clinic, bringing countless benefits to the city itself.

As the business grew, so did the need for expansion. In 1961, Wolfe Eye Clinic, now with four full-time physicians, moved into its current location on the east side of Marshalltown. By 1978, demand was surging, and an addition was connected to the building, significantly increasing the clinic's size, subspecialty areas and with Michael Hill, MD bringing back the previously discontinued ear, nose and throat surgery service. Dr. Russell Watt, the first non-Wolfe family ophthalmologist to join the clinic, wrote that the expansion was one of the biggest milestones in Wolfe Eye Clinic history.

"Substantial enlargement of the Marshalltown office to accommodate expanding ophthalmology and the additional specialty of ear, nose, and throat," he wrote in his notes. "This resulted in a tripling of the Clinic's size."

Even during expansion to other Iowa cities in the 1980s and '90s, most surgeons operated primarily in Marshalltown while they traveled to outlying branches on a rotating basis.

Also centrally located in Marshalltown is the corporate administrative and management team. This team works collaboratively with all offices around the state as well as with the board of directors. The following departments include insurance and billing, accounting, marketing and public relations, information technology, human resources, maintenance, and a centralized phone room for patient appointment scheduling. Physician services include cataract, glaucoma, corneal disease, LASIK consultations, optometry vitreoretinal consultations and laser surgeries, oculoplastic, pediatric ophthalmology as well as audiology.

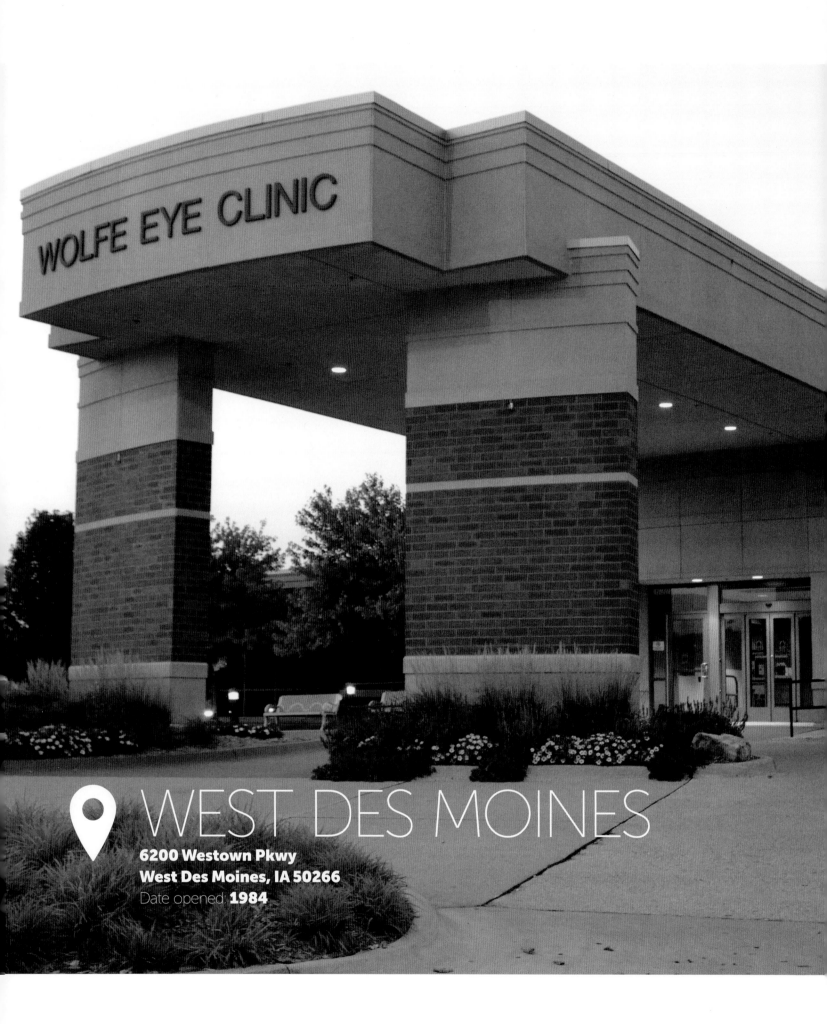

WEST DES MOINES

6200 Westown Pkwy
West Des Moines, IA 50266
Date opened: **1984**

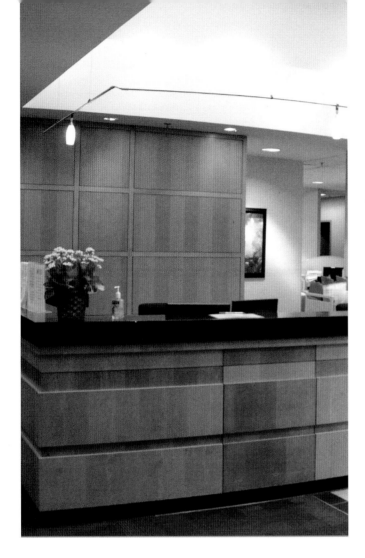

Providing services directly in Des Moines had been a goal for Wolfe Eye Clinic leadership since the early 1980s. It was the most populous city in Iowa, meaning there would be much more demand for the clinic's top-quality services. By the mid-1980s, about half of the patients traveling to Marshalltown came from the Greater Des Moines area. That presented both opportunity and obligation to better serve those patients.

In 1984, Wolfe Eye Clinic opened a satellite office in West Des Moines, and physicians drove from Marshalltown daily to examine and treat patients there. The office was in the Regency Building Complex on Westown Parkway just east of Interstate-35. They performed cataract surgical procedures at Charter Hospital near Merle Hay Mall.

Demand was slow. Dr. James Davison, who would often work in that first location, remembered there was plenty of downtime.

"We just weren't that busy because people just didn't know about us then," Davison said. "Fortunately, we had some terrific local optometrists who really desired our advanced surgical services for their patients, and they supported us well."

The practice grew because of these advanced procedures, like lens implants, small-incision surgery and laser surgery. These helped Wolfe Eye Clinic firmly establish itself in the Des Moines market. It took until 1991 for a full-time ophthalmologist to be placed in Des Moines — Dr. Steven Johnson — and from there, growth came quickly.

Over the years the Des Moines clinic has twice outgrown its facilities. In 1994 it moved to the West Lakes Complex on University Avenue, and 10 years later it moved to its current West Des Moines campus at 6200 Westown Parkway in West Des Moines on the west side of I-35.

In 2004, Wolfe Eye Clinic opened its very own 38,000 square foot, state-of-the-art building in West Des Moines, offering multiple ophthalmic subspecialty services to central Iowa patients. In 2007, Wolfe Eye Clinic incorporated a three operating room outpatient surgery center as part of a joint venture with Dallas County Hospital. In 2010, Wolfe assumed full ownership of the center but demand and growth ultimately exceeded its available space. So in 2019, that original center was closed as the new 25,000 square foot Wolfe Surgery Center building was opened. It sits as a companion building to the Clinic office building next door and houses state of the art technology including six operating rooms, the Des Moines Laser Center, Oculofacial Plastic Surgery Center and conference rooms.

Today, Wolfe Eye Clinic holds a majority market share in the Greater Des Moines metro. The West Des Moines clinic is the busiest of all the branches seeing an average of 265 patients per day in 2019. Optometrists and ophthalmologists throughout central Iowa refer complex medical and surgical patients for expert medical and surgical consultation services.

Another recent expansion in the West Des Moines market is the partnership with Children's Eye Clinic, which was founded in 1990 and was located in the nearby Lakeview Medical Park. The 2019 merger grew Wolfe Eye Clinic's pediatric ophthalmology services with the addition of Dr. Jean Spencer and her staff.

The West Des Moines Wolfe Eye Clinic is unparalleled in private ophthalmology practice in this portion of the Midwest. In 2019, it boasts a resident physician base of 13 ophthalmologists and five optometrists including subspecialists in cornea and external disease, refractive surgery, vitreoretinal disease and surgery, oculofacial plastics, glaucoma, and pediatrics and adult strabismus.

2019 was a busy year for Wolfe Eye Clinic because for better balanced patient convenience, it also opened an office on the Des Moines metro's east side in Pleasant Hill.

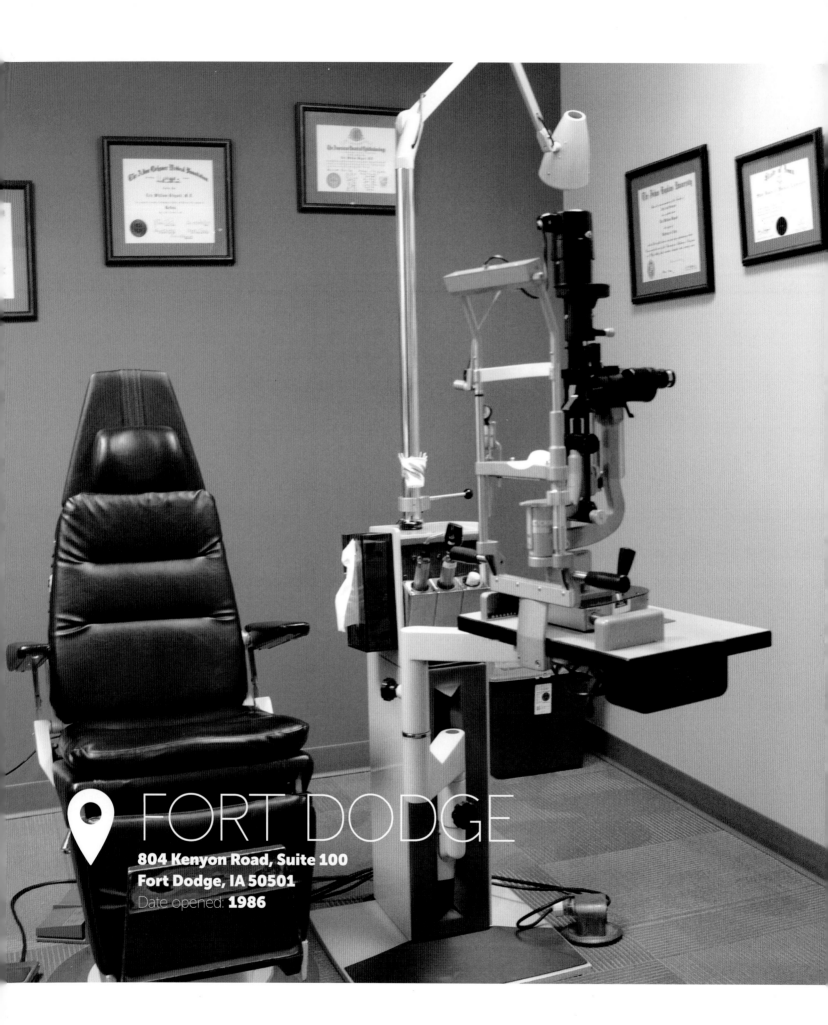

FORT DODGE

804 Kenyon Road, Suite 100
Fort Dodge, IA 50501
Date opened: **1986**

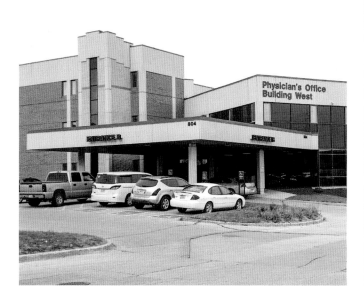

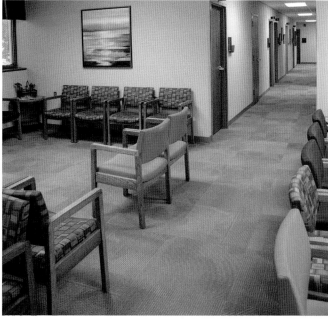

Fort Dodge represents a significant milestone in the history of Wolfe Eye Clinic. For one, it marked the second time Wolfe Eye Clinic consistently provided services outside of Marshalltown — the satellite office in West Des Moines was opened just two years before. Secondly, it helped launch an era of significant expansion for Wolfe Eye Clinic, which opened three new locations in five years.

During the early 1980s, expansion was often discussed among leadership. Thanks to Wolfe Eye Clinic's strong relationship with referring optometrists practicing in an Integrated model, leadership heard about an opportunity to open an office in Fort Dodge. The quality of ophthalmology surgery had been deficient in the area, and the local optometrists were clamoring for a local Wolfe Eye Clinic office where they could refer their patients.

There had been some surgical problems up there, and they wanted more competent services," said Dr. John Graether, who joined Wolfe Eye Clinic in 1962. "We were interested in expansion. And we had done a good job of developing a relationship with referring doctors, so they wanted us to come to Fort Dodge."

Wolfe Eye Clinic partnered with Fort Dodge Medical Center and took over a 4,000 square foot wing on the ground floor of the neighboring Medical Office Building. Initially the location wasn't staffed by a full-time ophthalmologist, meaning surgeons from Marshalltown made the regular trip up Interstate 35 and over on Highway 20 to serve patients on a rotating basis. The Marshalltown surgeons were rotating to the West Des Moines office already so they just added Fort Dodge to the schedule. According to a Fort Dodge Messenger report on the new location, the plan was to serve about 30 patients per day. And Wolfe Eye Clinic was welcomed with open arms.

Wolfe Eye Clinic still calls the hospital office building home, but it has significantly expanded its services. The first full-time ophthalmologist to serve Fort Dodge was Dr. Eric Bligard, who joined in 1987 and as of 2019 is still serving full time.

"In 1987, Fort Dodge badly needed an ophthalmologist and I needed a first job. It turned out to be a perfect marriage which is still in effect over 30 years later," Bligard said.

Today, there are eight subspecialty physicians who attend the location on a rotating basis. Services run the gamut, including cataract, glaucoma, cornea and external disease, LASIK, pediatric ophthalmology, oculoplastics as well as retina disease and retina surgery.

"We've been very lucky to have had Eric here for his entire career," Davison said. "He's been a wonderful asset to the community and remains a sound anchor and willing and versatile host for the rest of the crew that provides care in Fort Dodge."

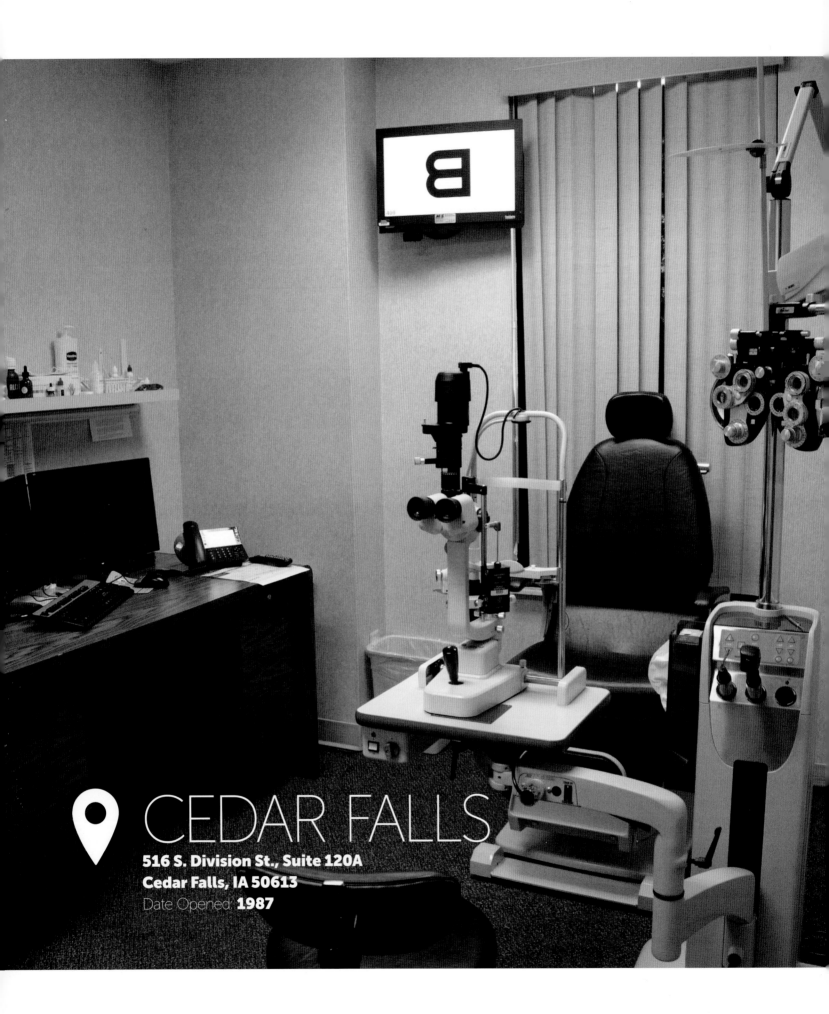

CEDAR FALLS

516 S. Division St., Suite 120A
Cedar Falls, IA 50613 —
Date Opened: **1987**

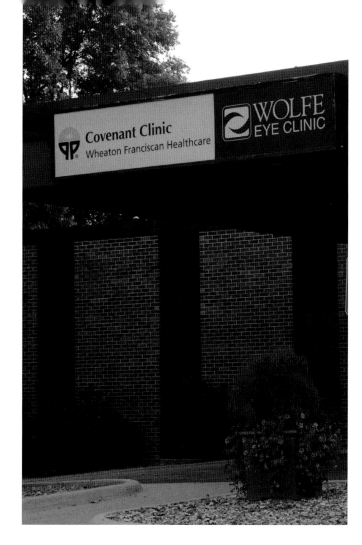

By the late 1980s, Wolfe Eye Clinic had already opened two separate locations beyond its home Marshalltown base — in West Des Moines and Fort Dodge. But those places had become successful satellite offices at the time, meaning physicians in Marshalltown had to travel to treat patients and were not based in either of those cites as full-time residents.

The location in Cedar Falls became the third satellite office.

In 1987, a group of six local Cedar Falls optometrists suggested Wolfe Eye Clinic move into the area. Patients already were traveling to Wolfe Eye Clinic in Marshalltown

because the standard of medical and surgical eye care in Cedar Falls was somewhat lacking. Wolfe Eye Clinic was welcomed by more new patients who were ready to receive a higher quality of care in their community. Physicians at Wolfe Eye Clinic were performing advanced eye surgeries not available in northeast Iowa at the time, so entering the market significantly raised the standard of care.

"They told us we should look in Cedar Falls because they still weren't doing the best intraocular lens implants and other more modern surgeries," said Dr. James Davison, who has been with Wolfe Eye Clinic since

1980. "So, we started our third satellite."

The first Cedar Falls office was located in a small three-room clinic at Sartori Hospital shared with the Wolfe ear, nose, throat (ENT) physicians who also traveled from Marshalltown to treat patients, Michael Hill, M.D. and Daniel Blum, M.D. By 1990, Wolfe Eye Clinic moved into an expanded Sartori Hospital professional building space where it had its own 6,000 square foot suite. Dr. Norman Woodlief and his family decided to move from Marshalltown to Cedar Falls to become a locally based full-time board-certified ophthalmologist and he was joined by three ophthalmic technicians and two nurses to provide full-time services. The move represented the second time Wolfe Eye Clinic placed full-time, on-site physicians outside of its Marshalltown home base.

"[Dr. John Graether, longtime physician with Wolfe Eye Clinic] said the additional space, staff and equipment in the new office soon will allow Wolfe Eye Clinic doctors to handle a wide range of laser procedures, to treat disorders of the retina, the innermost portion of the eye," read a report in the May 31,

1990 Cedar Falls-Waterloo Courier.

Wolfe Eye Clinic continues to operate in the Sartori professional building today with six subspecialty physicians who care for patients on an ongoing weekly rotational basis, three of whom call Cedar Falls home. Services include comprehensive ophthalmology with specialists in LASIK, cataract, glaucoma, medical and cosmetic oculoplastics as well as retina disease and surgery. Some of the original area optometrists that requested Wolfe to open a clinic in Cedar Falls have moved to work in the adjacent suite while Wolfe surgeons still work closely with optometrists from all around the Cedar Valley region.

"I moved to Cedar Falls directly out of residency in Miami, Florida and the area has far exceeded my expectations," said Dr. Benjamin Mason, one of the ophthalmologists based in Cedar Falls. "It is truly a wonderful community and a great place to raise a family."

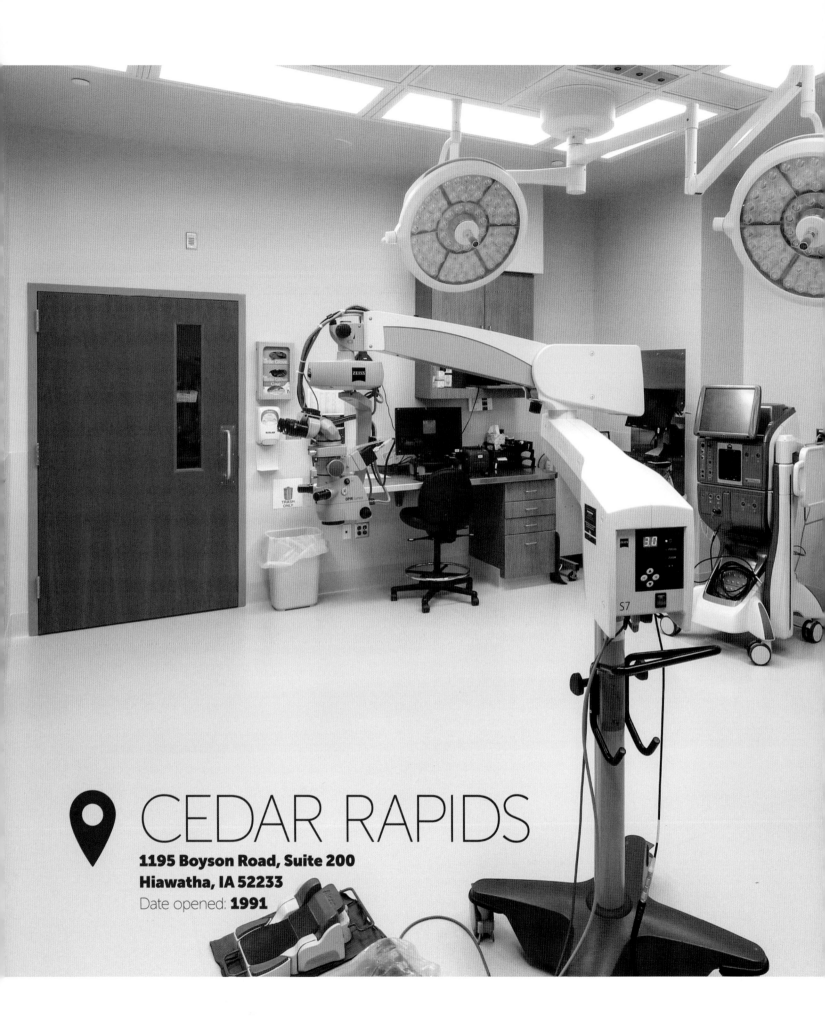

CEDAR RAPIDS

1195 Boyson Road, Suite 200
Hiawatha, IA 52233
Date opened: **1991**

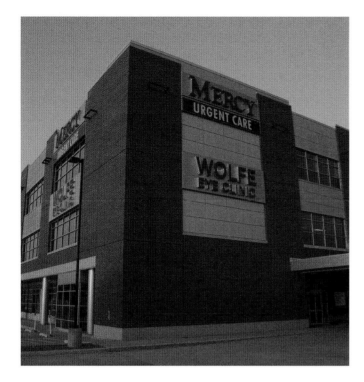

The expansion to Cedar Rapids wasn't the most extravagant, but it was crucial to the growth of the Wolfe Eye Clinic business. In 1991, Wolfe Eye Clinic opened a location in a small, white house in Cedar Rapids. Reception was placed in what used to be a living room. Exam rooms were placed in various bedrooms. The doctor's office/break room was in a bedroom next to the only bathroom.

Despite the tight space, Wolfe Eye Clinic's top-notch service took off and grew quickly. The medical surgical cutting-edge eye care procedures drew significant demand, which created an unintended consequence for physicians. Most doctors were located in Marshalltown, but they traveled across the state to provide services in new offices.

Cedar Rapids was another location to balance.

Looking back now, it was rather exciting and challenging at the same time.

"You'd have one plate, then you'd start spinning it, and then another one would slow down, so you'd have to spin it again and add another," Dr. James Davison said with a laugh. "We had all these plates spinning."

Dr. Todd Gothard was the first Wolfe Eye Clinic physician based in Cedar Rapids, joining the practice in 1993. At this time, Gothard was the first cornea subspecialist to serve the Cedar Rapids and Cedar Falls patient areas.

There was some initial pushback by local ophthalmologists when the clinic moved into the area,

and there were even discussions of shutting down the Cedar Rapids branch early in its tenure. But Wolfe Eye Clinic stuck it out.

"I remember sitting in [our board room] deciding whether we were going to stay in Cedar Rapids or not," said Dr. John Graether, who joined Wolfe Eye Clinic in 1962. "We decided it was foolish to abandon such a good patient service area."

In due time, demand significantly outgrew the space. In 1996, services were moved across the street into a new 8,000 square foot facility which was only half occupied until in 1997, when Wolfe Eye Clinic brought on Dr. Charles Barnes as the first vitreoretinal surgeon in the metro area. Two full-time physicians were placed in Cedar Rapids, reducing the amount of "plate spinning" for Marshalltown-based ophthalmologists.

Since that time several other eye care specialists have been added into a rotation not only for cataract surgery, corneal procedures and retina disease, but glaucoma treatments, pediatric and adult

strabismus evaluation as well as LASIK surgeries.

Providing these additional subspecialty patient care services created growing pains because of the lack of adequate space for treatment and testing. Therefore, in 2017 in collaboration with Mercy Medical Center, the clinic moved into a new 22,800 square foot medical facility located conveniently off Interstate 380 in Hiawatha. This new facility not only provided much needed clinical and testing needs, but patients could have their outpatient eye care surgery procedures accomplished in the same building, making this an easy two-step process for patients. This office also became home to a state-of-the-art climate-controlled LASIK laser surgery suite serving eastern Iowa. Services in Hiawatha (Cedar Rapids) include cataracts, glaucoma, cornea, LASIK, pediatrics, strabismus and retina disease management and surgery.

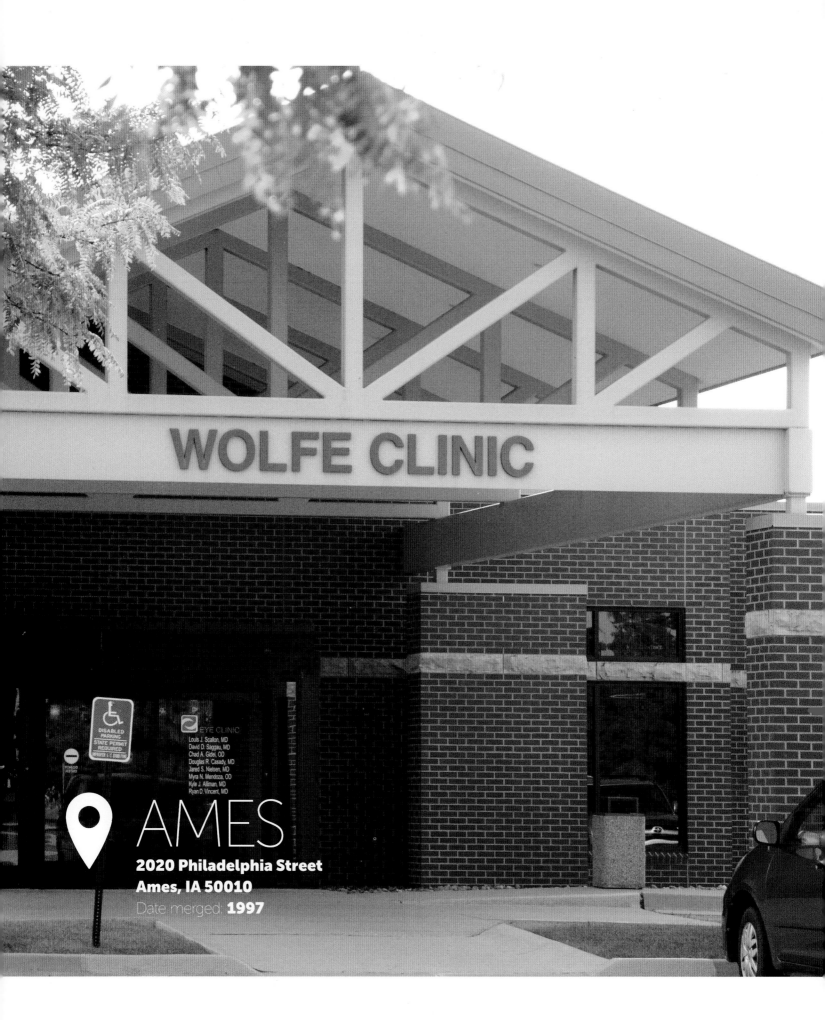

EYE CLINIC

Louis J. Scallon, MD
David D. Saggau, MD
Chad A. Gidel, OD
Douglas R. Casady, MD
Jared S. Nielsen, MD
Myra N. Mendoza, OD
Kyle J. Alliman, MD
Ryan D. Vincent, MD

AMES

2020 Philadelphia Street
Ames, IA 50010
Date merged: **1997**

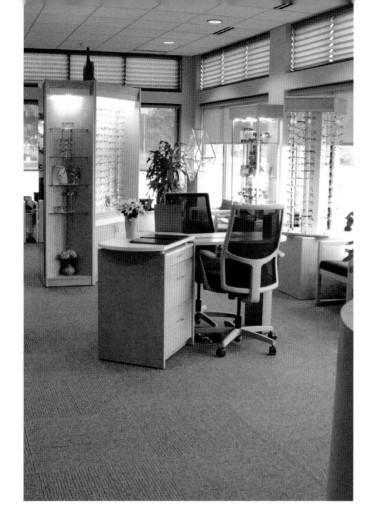

In the mid-1990s there was another eye clinic located approximately 35 miles west of Marshalltown in Ames, Iowa, operating with a mission similar to that of Wolfe Eye Clinic's. The physicians at Iowa Eye Care Physicians, P.C., practiced a high standard of patient care, a similar business model and maintained a deep care for the community. Wolfe Eye Clinic, which embodied all of these important values, decided to approach the Ames business about joining together.

"We had worked with them before," said Dr. James Davison, who joined Wolfe Eye Clinic in 1980. "They had wonderful people. Eventually we continued talking with these guys and found that we had really everything in common with their philosophy and how they liked to treat patients and work with optometrists. We all realized that, together we would be happier partners of a better enterprise."

Iowa Eye Care Physicians was also performing cutting-edge surgeries, just like Wolfe Eye Clinic. They had a strong administrative team in place headed by their long time administrator, Randy Eckard. In the course of discussions, Dr. Dean Harms, Dr. Daniel Vos and Dr. Louis Scallon realized that working with Wolfe Eye Clinic would still allow them to uphold their patient-centric approach while creating efficiencies and provide a much broader level of subspecialty eye care to their patients in Ames and their other outreach clinic sites.

On Feb 1, 1997, Wolfe Eye Clinic's administrative team was made even stronger with the addition of Randy Eckard as Chief Operating Officer through the successful merger with Iowa Eye Care Physicians.

"Randy was an imaginative and tireless COO and a great contributor to the future growth of the Clinic and stayed on with us until his retirement in 2019.," said Dr. James Davison.

The merger was a huge boost to citizens in both the Ames area and other Wolfe Eye Clinic locations, expanding its geographical footprint in central Iowa.

"The late 1990's was a time of significant change in health care," said Scallon, current Wolfe Eye Clinic surgeon. "Smaller single-specialty groups such as ours were looking for ways to become more efficient and broaden the services which we could provide to our patients. Joining Wolfe Eye Clinic enabled us to achieve these goals. It has been great to be part of a forward-thinking group which is committed to providing the highest standard of eye care."

In 2001, the merged clinic moved from its original free-standing building location (established in 1976) across from Mary Greeley Medical Center, and opened a new, 13,500 sq ft. Wolfe Eye Clinic Ames office building located on the northeast side of the city. The new office was easily accessible off the interstate making it more convenient for patients who were traveling from out of town to access services.

Today, the Ames location is one of the largest in the Wolfe Eye Clinic system offering complete medical and surgical eye care, including cataract, glaucoma, retinal disease, corneal disease, LASIK evaluations, pediatrics and medical and cosmetic oculoplastics. Using the latest medical and surgical technologies and eye care treatments, the board-certified subspecialists at Wolfe Eye Clinic, along with its staff, provide the highest possible standard of eye care excellence for the people of central Iowa.

Wolfe Eye Clinic in Waterloo is housed in what used be a bank. The building was still outfitted with drive-thru deposit boxes when physicians moved in, in 2000. Dr. James Davison remembers, with a grin, quipping about how physicians could revolutionize speed of patient service.

"They still had the little boxes where you drive up to the bank and put stuff for deposit," he said. "We'd joke that patients could stick their heads in there, get their surgery done and drive away."

Jokes aside, demand was strong in the Cedar Valley area, and the clinic's Waterloo residents enjoyed the easy access to the clinic on the south side of town, just off of the Highway 20 exit, making it convenient access for patients. Located on the first level, the main area of patient exam rooms displays a large window that looks out onto the fourth green at Sunnyside Country Club, which can make it hard to stay inside on warm days.

Wolfe Eye Clinic's decision to move into the Waterloo area complemented the successful patient friendly Cedar Falls location, which had been in operation for over a decade. Both offices were able to share an expanded level of multi-specialty eye care providers to a broader geographic group of patients.

Today, six physicians staff the Waterloo clinic, providing comprehensive ophthalmology care, LASIK consultations, and evaluation and surgery for glaucoma, corneal disease, pediatric eye conditions, cataracts and retina diseases.

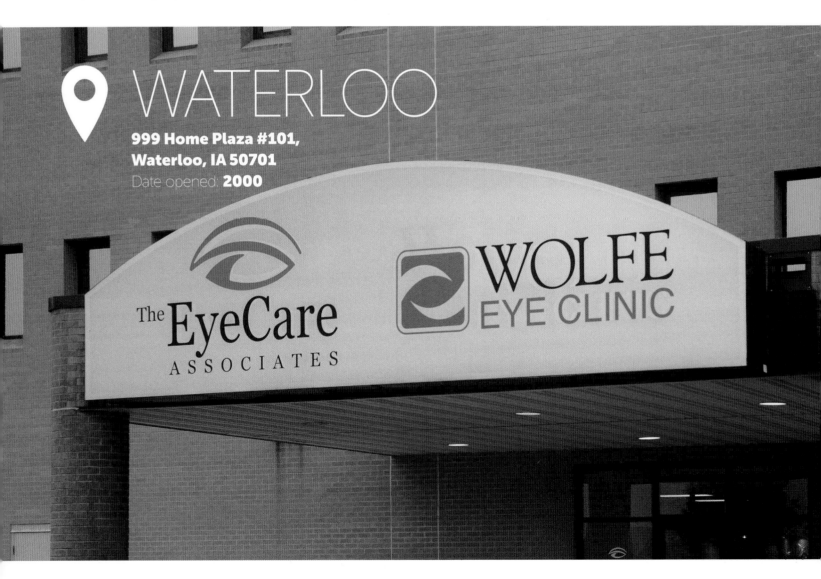

WATERLOO

999 Home Plaza #101, Waterloo, IA 50701
Date opened: **2000**

The EyeCare ASSOCIATES

WOLFE EYE CLINIC

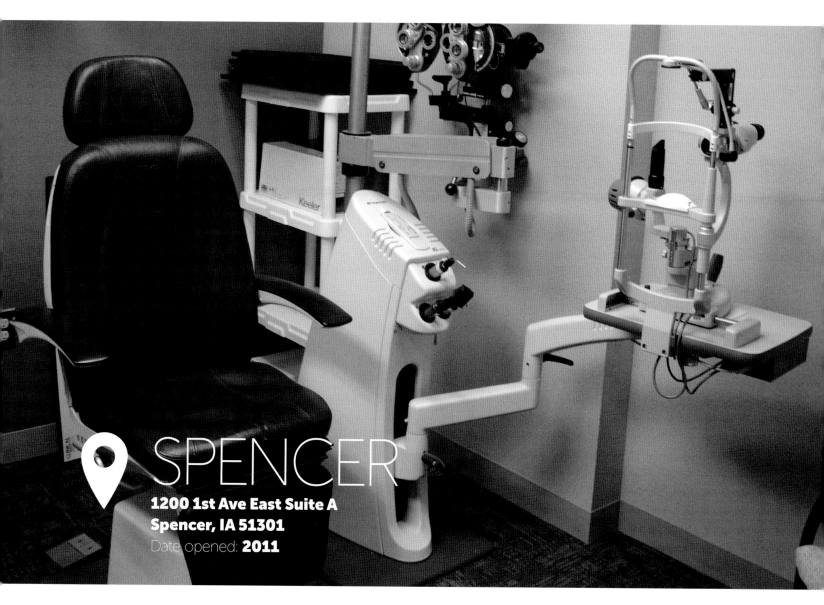

SPENCER

1200 1st Ave East Suite A
Spencer, IA 51301
Date opened: **2011**

Wolfe Eye Clinic had been serving communities in northwest Iowa since the early 1990s by providing cataract surgery at outreach locations in Estherville, Emmetsburg and Algona. However, in 2011, Spencer Municipal Hospital, along with area optometrists, asked Wolfe Eye Clinic to consider opening a permanent main office. Having a full-time eye surgeon would allow for better, more convenient access for patients, and would complement and improve the quality of eye care that was being provided in the northwest Iowa region. Previously, Fort Dodge was the most northwest of Wolfe Eye Clinic's main locations.

The office, which is located within the Spencer Municipal Hospital medical campus, allowed Wolfe Eye Clinic to further serve northwest Iowa patients as well as individuals from as far as Sioux Falls, South Dakota and Southern Minnesota. Dr. Stephen Fox, who joined the clinic in 2008 and had been previously based in the Fort Dodge office, was delighted to provide full-time ophthalmic services in Spencer when it opened in 2011 and still serves this office today as a cataract surgeon and general ophthalmologist. Fox had always been passionate for helping patients in rural communities and felt privileged to be a part of providing these important surgical services.

"Dr. Fox is just a great person, and we had a great place for him," Dr. James Davison said. "It was a wonderful match for him and the community. And he and his staff are such terrific hosts to all of the visiting surgical teams."

Today, several other surgeons rotate through visiting the Spencer office to provide care closer to home for patients. Medical eye care services include cataract evaluation and surgery, retina disease and surgery, glaucoma and corneal disease.

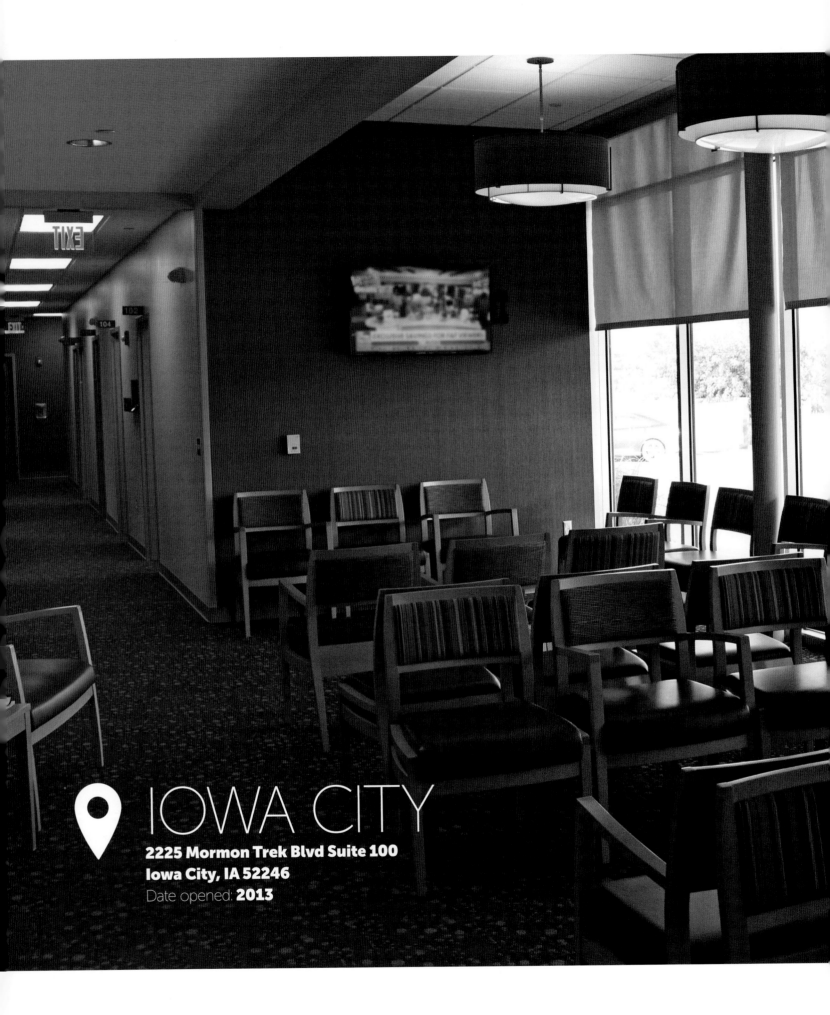

IOWA CITY

2225 Mormon Trek Blvd Suite 100
Iowa City, IA 52246
Date opened: **2013**

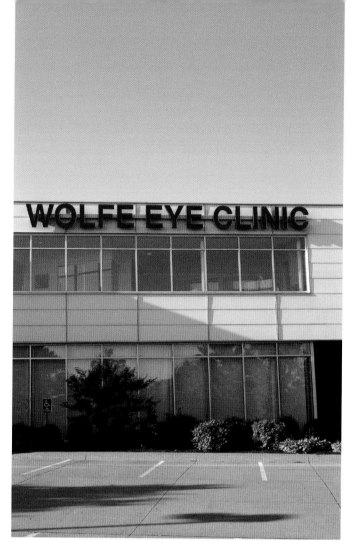

Iowa City has more physicians per captia than anywhere else in Iowa. The University of Iowa College of Medicine educates about 50% of the state's doctors, and several Wolfe Eye Clinic surgeons started their medical training at the University of Iowa College of Medicine Department of Ophthalmology due to its highly regarded and impressive national ranking.

Starting in the late 1990s, the clinic began sending an ophthalmologist from the Cedar Rapids office into an existing Iowa City private optometry practice to see referred patients on a part-time basis. In 2013, Wolfe Eye Clinic decided to expand into Iowa City to further its reach in eastern Iowa by opening a fully equipped office of its own. The local Iowa City region optometrists as well as those from further southeast Iowa had asked Wolfe Eye Clinic to open a clinic in the area to provide them an alternative to refer subspecialty eye care with

easy access. Wolfe Eye Clinic jumped in and has seen success ever since.

"We've done well there, and we've been able to expand," said Dr. John Graether, who started with Wolfe Eye Clinic in 1962, is now retired and encouraged leadership to get into Iowa City. "That market was just so important, and it was important for us to have a presence there and to better serve patients from southeast Iowa."

The location is housed in a beautiful building, clad with modern white walls and windows. Services include cataract, retina and corneal disease evaluation and treatment, as well as evaluation for LASIK laser vision correction surgery. The physician team in Iowa City has played a large role in helping Wolfe Eye Clinic lead the way in eye care for Iowans with their dedication to peer research and investing in the best technology for all patients.

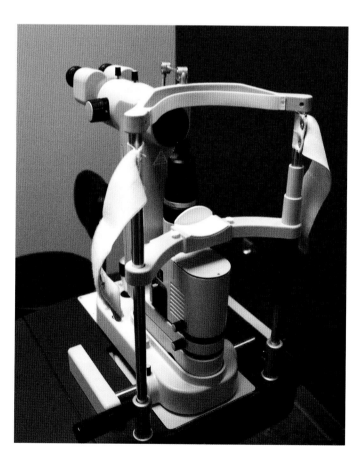

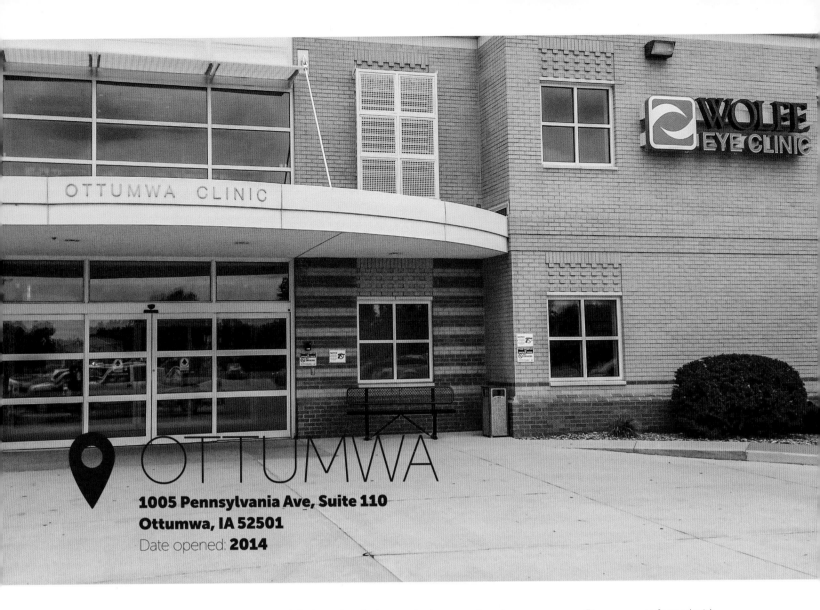

OTTUMWA

1005 Pennsylvania Ave, Suite 110
Ottumwa, IA 52501
Date opened: **2014**

The history of how Wolfe Eye Clinic moved into Ottumwa starts in 1983, when southeast Iowa Eye Specialists began under Dr. Norman Hutchison. Dr. Gregory Thorgaard joined the practice, followed by Dr. Mariannette Miller-Meeks, and together, the three ophthalmologists merged with an optometry practice headed by Dr. R. Payson Moreland, Family Eye Care, in 1998 to form a collaborative group of providers that made up Heartland Eye Care.

Located in rural southeast Iowa, and with Dr. Hutchison facing retirement, the doctors reached out to Wolfe Eye Clinic regarding a potential merger. While discussions had been ongoing for more than a decade, Heartland Eye Care was experiencing an increasing demand for expanded eye care services. Along with that, there was difficulty in recruiting physicians to rural Iowa, which made all the more sense to continue discussions with Wolfe Eye Clinic in the years leading up to 2014.

Dr. James Davison, who was integral in both the Ames and Ottumwa mergers, believed the merger to be mutually beneficial — expanding staffing resources for clinic operations and increasing access to eye care subspecialists for patients in southeast Iowa. Additionally, both groups shared a common mission of providing excellence in patient care.

"These folks were really terrific, and they wanted to do the right thing by their patients," Davison said. "These were the kind of people that we've always wanted, so it was really a natural fit. It was especially good because it continued our founding tradition of surgeons and optometrists working shoulder to shoulder together."

In 2014, the merger was completed, and it expanded Wolfe Eye Clinic's reach to southeast Iowa. It was an exciting time for both staffs.

"A merger was formed with Wolfe Eye Clinic to help broaden the services offered to our patients," Thorgaard said when the merger was announced. "Combining the practices allowed access to additional subspecialty care for our patients, close to home."

Ottumwa services include general ophthalmological care, evaluation and medical treatment of cataracts, cornea disease, glaucoma, oculofacial plastic conditions, and retina disease. LASIK eye surgery consultations and family optometry with optical services are also available at the Ottumwa clinic.

Constructed with the intention of expanding Wolfe Eye Clinic's services in the Des Moines metro area, the Pleasant Hill location is one of the newest offices. The decision to expand with a satellite office in the Greater Des Moines east side had several benefits. With the retina service continuing to expand its services due to high patient demand, it was becoming increasing difficult to accommodate timely services in West Des Moines.

Demographic studies showed that there was an increasing number of patients driving to the West Des Moines office from the east and southeast corners of the state. The east side office expansion allowed for easier patient access, more appointment availability to serve patients and a relief of space in the West Des Moines office.

Equally important, the newest Pleasant Hill office is now used to deliver the services of other subspecialty eye care providers, most of which travel from the West Des Moines office.

Services include evaluation and treatment for cataracts, corneal disease, glaucoma and retina. LASIK laser vision correction evaluations are also offered at the Pleasant Hill location.

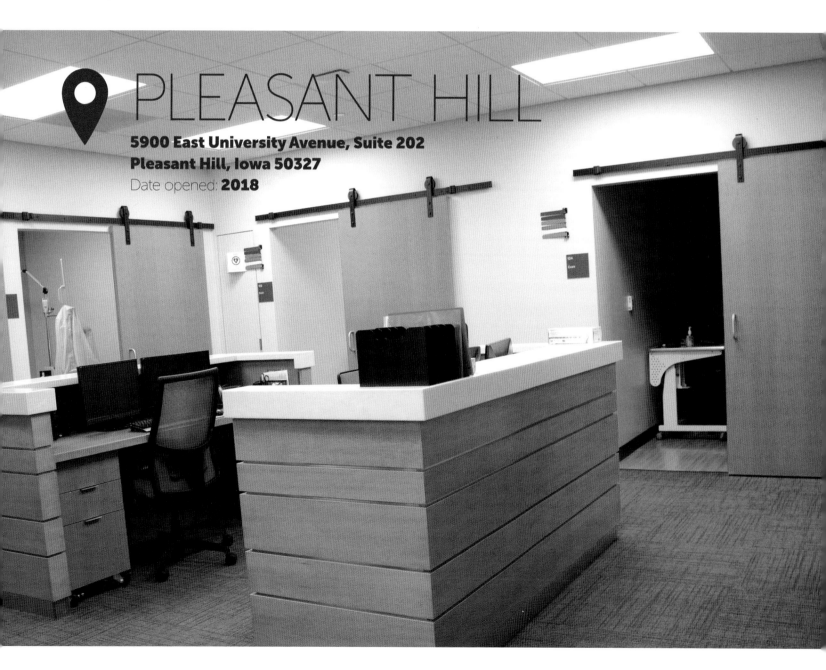

PLEASANT HILL

5900 East University Avenue, Suite 202
Pleasant Hill, Iowa 50327
Date opened: **2018**

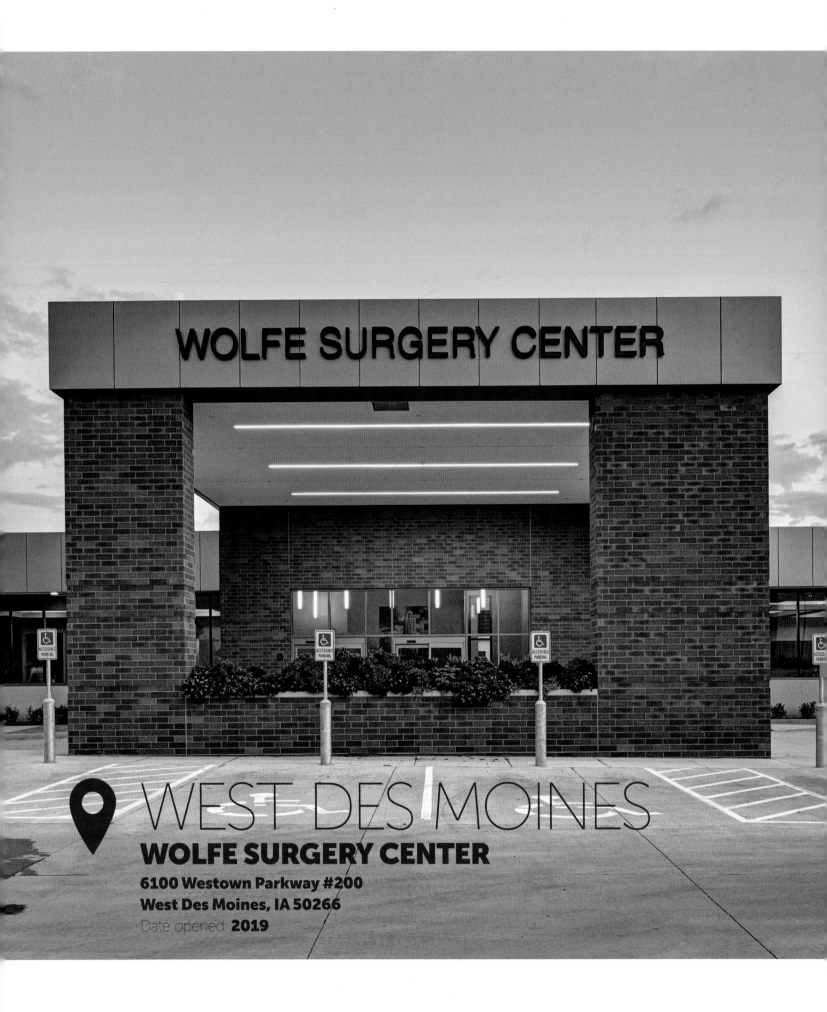

WEST DES MOINES
WOLFE SURGERY CENTER

6100 Westown Parkway #200
West Des Moines, IA 50266

Date opened: **2019**

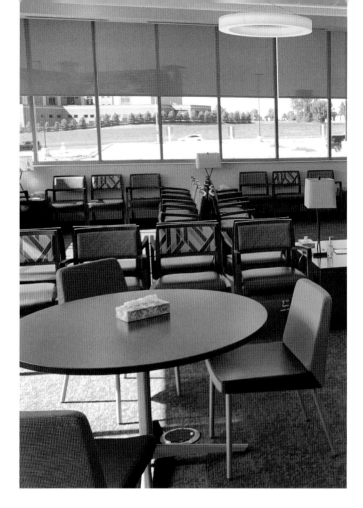

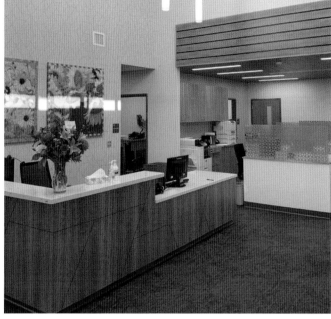

When Wolfe Eye Clinic built its current West Des Moines office in 2004, plans were in place to create a surgery center on part of the lower level of the clinic. However, there was a legal requirement: Iowa state law dictated that any surgery center needed approval for a Certificate of Need. The best way to gain approval was an affiliation with a local hospital already providing outpatient surgical services.

In light of the great demand for ophthalmic surgery in the Des Moines area, Wolfe Eye Clinic approached Dallas County Hospital. The clinic property was located in Dallas County, just west of the Polk County line. A partnership with the

hospital would be beneficial to both entities and the public. The hospital agreed, and surgery center construction of the three-operating room center was completed in 2007. In 2010, Wolfe Eye Clinic purchased full ownership of the surgical suite and named it the Wolfe Surgery Center.

Seven years later, the Wolfe Surgery Center had outgrown its limited space. There was a pressing need to expand the number of operating rooms so more patients could be served in a timely manner. The clinic needed more space, too.

"We had to do something," said Dr. James Davison, one of the premier ophthalmic surgeons in the Midwest. "We thought,

'Let's build something that we could grow into.'"

Fortunately, through thoughtful foresight by the board, Wolfe Eye Clinic had retained additional land next to the current clinic, which was a convenient, close-by location for a new surgery center.

"We built a beautiful companion building whose appearance matched the clinic building." Davison said. "So then we had a campus."

An expanded state-of-the-art 25,000 square foot ambulatory surgery center, housing six operating rooms, laser center, cosmetic surgery center and conference rooms was created. The new facility

opened in 2019 and is the largest dedicated ophthalmic surgery center in the Midwest. It serves patients eye care needs throughout the region.

"It's a dream come true," Davison said. "It's huge, and it's really one of the most beautiful centers you will find in the country. I've never seen anything as contemporary as this that provides such state-of-the-art care. I'm thrilled every time I walk in there."

Wolfe Surgery Center serves patients undergoing many types of eye procedures, including cataract, retina, cornea, strabismus, facial oculoplastics, glaucoma, LASIK and more.

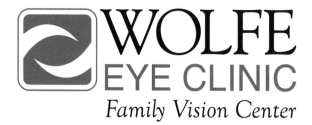

FAMILY VISION CENTERS

Since the beginning, the physicians of Wolfe Eye Clinic have worked in partnership with the many optometrists across Iowa taking care of patients together. When a person needs advanced medical eye care, or surgical intervention, these referral relationships ensure seamless care between a patient's primary care optometrist and surgeons at Wolfe Eye Clinic.

Mainly located in rural areas, Wolfe Family Vision Centers are an important part of the Wolfe Eye Clinic business model. Like their peers, these Wolfe-affiliated optometrists provide primary family eye care and are essential in the communities they serve. They provide comprehensive family eye exams, are experts in contact lenses and offer a large selection of fashionable eye wear. They also treat eye injuries and infections and diagnose and manage many ocular disorders including cataracts, glaucoma, macular degeneration and diabetic eye disease, using Wolfe Eye Clinic surgeons for advanced medical and surgical referrals.

Wolfe Family Vision Centers started in the late 1990s and have grown over the years to nine locations.

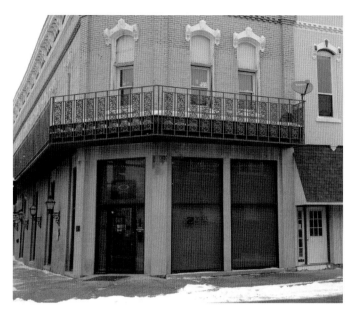

Albia

101 Benton Ave E. Albia, IA 52531

Located in the heart of Albia, east of Main Street and off Benton Avenue, the Albia clinic opened in 2014 as part of the Wolfe Eye Clinic and Heartland Eye Care merger in Ottumwa. Dr. R. Payson Moreland purchased the Albia practice from Dr. Gene Wolski in 1997 and later merged it into Heartland Eye Care when he joined Dr. Gregory Thorgaard and Dr. Norman Hutchison in 1998.

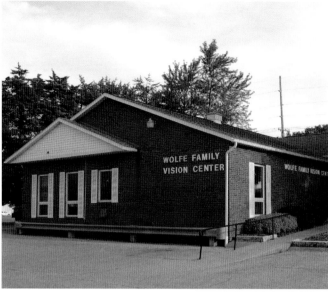

Fairfield

100 S 23rd St. Fairfield, IA 52556

Established in 1996, the Fairfield clinic was the first Wolfe Family Vision Center. Throughout the years, optometrists Dr. Joseph Johll, Dr. Patricia Blume and Dr. Kreg Harper provided care to the residents of Fairfield and surrounding communities. For the past 7 years, Dr. Daniel Sliwinski has continued the tradition, providing care to new generations of Iowans throughout southeast Iowa.

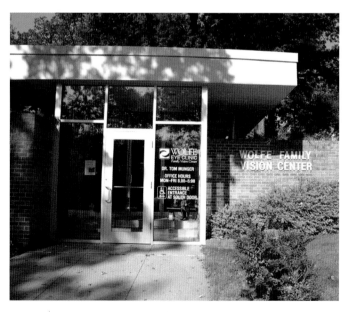

Sac City

202 S 6th St. Sac City, IA 50583

The Sac City clinic was acquired in 2002 from Dr. Thomas Munger. Located in the county seat of Sac County, just one block south of historic Main Street, this clinic was the first Wolfe Family Vision Center established for residents living in western Iowa. Today, it continues to provide comprehensive eye exams, treatment for eye infections and injuries and eye disease management and treatment.

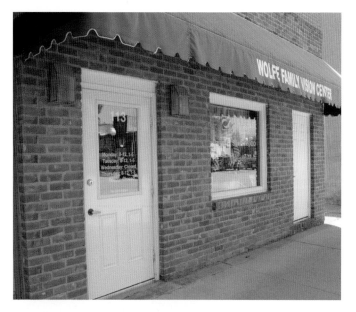

Sigourney

113 E Marion St. Sigourney, IA 52591

The establishment of the Sigourney clinic in 2004 welcomed Dr. Jerry Gibson to the Wolfe Eye Clinic family. After his retirement, doctors based in the nearby Fairfield clinic began visiting Sigourney. This clinic, located in Sigourney's historic square, serves the residents of Keokuk County and surrounding areas.

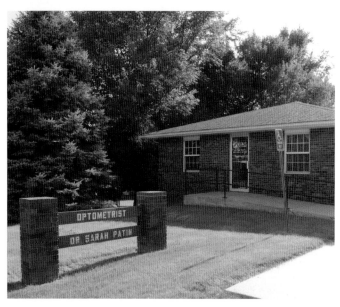

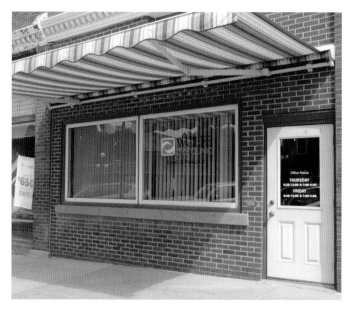

Toledo

1302 S Broadway St. Toledo, IA 52342

Traer

524 2nd St. Traer, IA 50675

The Toledo and Traer clinics were acquired in 1999 from Dr. Marshall Walker, who continued to serve these communities until retiring in 2015. Since then, Dr. Sarah Patin has continued providing primary family eye care in these offices for Iowans throughout Tama County and surrounding areas.

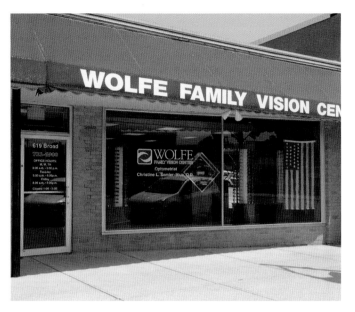

Story City

619 Broad St. Story City, IA 50248

The Story City clinic was acquired in 2004 from Dr. Christine Semler, who continues to serve the community today. This clinic, located in the heart of Story City, helps people throughout the community see better by providing primary eye care services including comprehensive eye exams for children and adults, treatment for eye injuries and infections and eye disease management.

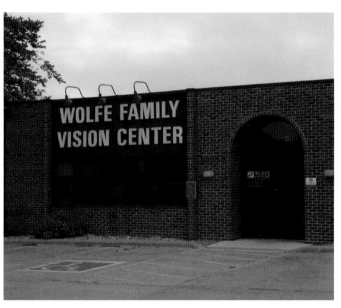

Waverly

2020 3rd Ave NW B. Waverly, IA 50677

The Waverly clinic was acquired from Dr. Todd Verdon in 1998. Upon his retirement in 2003, Dr. Mark Jeppesen joined and has been there ever since. Located on the north side of town, just a few blocks from Wartburg College, this clinic serves Iowans throughout northeast Iowa.

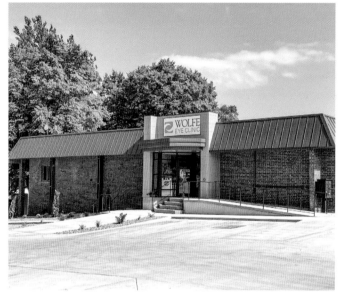

Webster City

1620 Superior St. #3 Webster City, IA 50595

The Webster City clinic opened in 1998, adding Dr. Robert Nieman and Dr. James Tesdahl to the Wolfe family, followed shortly by Dr. John Ferrell in 2000. For many years, the clinic was located on Division Street, on the north side of town. In 2019, the clinic moved south onto Superior Street, closer to Highway 20. At twice the size, the new location allows doctors to care for even more residents in north-central Iowa.

OUTREACH LOCATIONS

In an effort to provide greater access for patients, Wolfe Eye Clinic proudly partners with optometrists and hospitals across the state of Iowa to bring high-quality services in a more convenient manner, closer to home.

The idea of outreach partnerships was conceived in the early 1990s when CEO Kevin Swartz and clinic leadership wished to find new ways to reach underserved communities around the state. At the time, advancements in cataract surgery techniques had evolved and surgery could now be performed as an outpatient procedure. With numerous rural towns not having surgical eye services within many miles, these collaborations were a great way to provide increased access and care.

"We come in and we can serve patients locally," Swartz said.

"We can keep the patient close to home by working with local optometrists and hospitals. Wolfe Eye Clinic's Iowa and community-centered approach filled a need."

The first outreach sites were established in West Union, Estherville and Newton. Today, Wolfe cataract surgeons serve nearly 30 outreach locations, touching almost every part of Iowa. Physicians and their staff travel hundreds of miles every week to bring expert services and quality care to these communities.

ALGONA
Kossuth Regional Health
Center 1515 South Phillips St.
Algona, IA 50511

BOONE
Boone County Hospital
1015 Union St.
Boone, IA 50036

CHARITON
Lucas County Health Center
1200 N. 7th St.
Chariton, IA 50049

CHEROKEE
**Regional Health Services
of Howard County**
235 Eighth Ave. West
Cresco, IA 52136

CRESCO
**Regional Health Services
of Howard County**
235 8th Ave W,
Cresco, IA 52136

CRESTON
**Greater Regional
Medical Center**
1700 W. Townline St.
Creston, IA 50801

EMMETSBURG
Palo Alto County Hospital
3201 First St.
Emmetsburg, IA 50536

ESTHERVILLE
Avera Holy Family Hospital
826 N. Eighth Street
Estherville, IA 51334

GRINNELL
Grinnell Regional Medical Center
210 4th Ave,
Grinnell, IA 50112

GRUNDY CENTER
**Grundy County
Memorial Hospital**
201 East J Ave.
Grundy Center, IA 50638

HAMPTON
Franklin General Hospital
1720 Central Ave.
East Hampton, IA 50441

INDIANOLA
**MercyOne Indianola Family
Medicine**
2006 N 4th St Ste 200
Indianola, IA 50125

IOWA FALLS
Hansen Family Hospital
920 South Oak St.
Iowa Falls, IA 50126

JEFFERSON
Greene County Medical Center
1000 West Lincoln Way
Jefferson, IA 50129

KNOXVILLE
Knoxville Hospital & Clinics
1002 S. Lincoln St.
Knoxville, IA 50138

LAKE CITY
Stewart Memorial Hospital
1301 W Main St.
Lake City, IA 51449

NEVADA
Story County Medical Center
640 South 19th Street
Nevada, IA 50201

NEW HAMPTON
**MercyOne New Hampton Medical
Center**
308 N Maple Ave.
New Hampton, IA 50659

NEWTON
Skiff Medical Center
204 N 4th Ave. E
Newton, IA 50208

OSCEOLA
Clark County Hospital
800 South Fillmore
Osceola, IA 50213

OSKALOOSA
**Mahaska Health Hospital &
Family Care Clinic**
1229 C Ave E.
Oskaloosa, IA 52577

PELLA
Pella Regional Hospital
404 Jefferson Street
Pella, IA 50219

PERRY
Dallas County Hospital
610 10th St.
Perry, IA 50220

SPIRIT LAKE
Lakes Regional Healthcare
2323 Highway 71 South
Spirit Lake, IA 51360

STORM LAKE
**Buena Vista Regional
Medical Center**
1525 W 5th St,
Storm Lake, IA 50588, USA

WASHINGTON
**Name Washington County
Hospital and Clinic**
400 E Polk St.
Washington, IA 52353

WEST UNION
Palmer Lutheran Health Center
112 W Jefferson St.
West Union, IA 52175

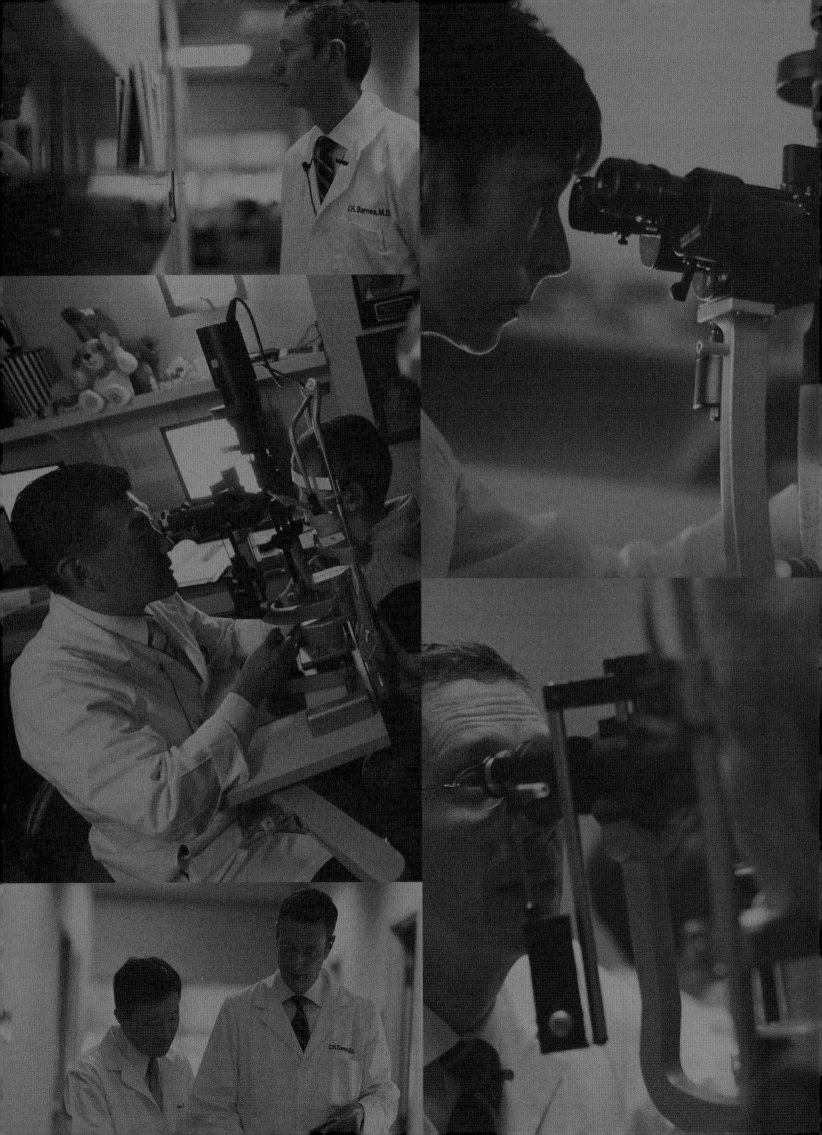

IOWA'S MOST
TRUSTED

Medical + Surgical

Eye Specialists

WOLFE EYE CLINIC

Founding Fathers

OTIS R. WOLFE, M.D.

CATARACT EVALUATION AND SURGERY

FOUNDED WOLFE EYE CLINIC: 1919

LOCATION: Marshalltown

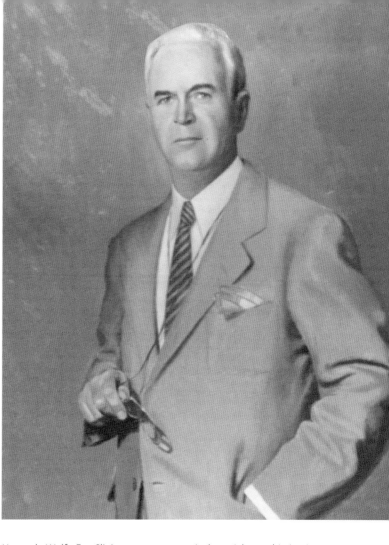

Dr. Otis R. Wolfe was always thinking ahead. A trained optometrist and ophthalmologist in his home state of Kansas, Otis R. moved to Chicago during World War I to train under prominent ear, eye, nose and throat doctors there. After expressing a desire to start a business of his own, Wolfe founded Wolfe Eye Clinic in Marshalltown in 1919 in part because of its central Iowa location and access to the railroad. The founding of Wolfe Eye Clinic revolutionized cataract care in the Midwest and throughout the United States in the 1920s and '30s.

Wolfe was dedicated to helping as many people as possible. He partnered with optometrists to extend care into more communities, sparking controversy within the ophthalmic profession. He started the Wolfe Foundation in 1936 to help bring eye care to those in need and fund critical research to advance surgical science.

His completion of one of the first Barraquer method cataract surgeries in the United States advanced the industry in immeasurable ways. The Barraquer method of removing a cataract was developed by Dr. Ignacio Barraquer in Barcelona, Spain. Wolfe always looked for the next best treatment option, and that's what ascended Wolfe Eye Clinic to new heights.

He made Wolfe Eye Clinic a national leader in ophthalmic services and handed it over to his sons Otis D. and Russell, both ophthalmologists, and Henry, an optometrist, who helped grow the business even further. Wolfe was the individual behind the innovative mindset at Wolfe Eye Clinic in its founding years.

A big part of his legacy today is the introduction of something quite radical at the time but is now hailed as perhaps the best method of modern eye-care practice. It's the integrated care model, where ophthalmologists and optometrists practice together in a system of communities, shoulder to shoulder to improve access to care and provide medical and surgical specialty sophistication to all who might need it.

After his death in 1954, an optometry industry publication wrote a glowing obituary. In it, Wolfe was painted as a man who changed eye care for the better. "Dr. Wolfe never allowed professional differences to stand between the man and the work to which his life was dedicated," the publication read. "He worked for the benefit of mankind, regardless of the professional implications. ... The field of visual care has been considerably enriched by his life."

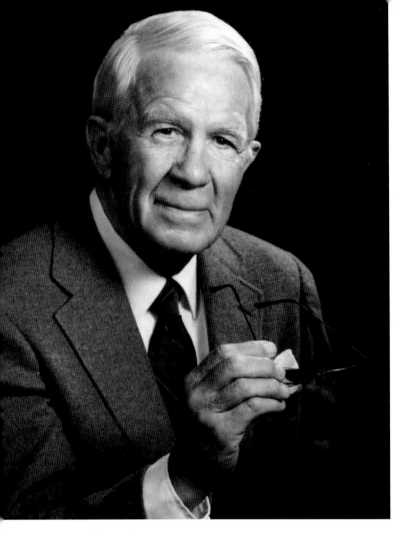

OTIS D. WOLFE, M.D.

CATARACT EVALUATION AND SURGERY

JOINED WOLFE EYE CLINIC: 1946

LOCATION: Marshalltown

The oldest of the Wolfe sons, Dr. Otis D. Wolfe, affectionately known as "Otey," had an innovative mind. He was born in Palco, Kansas, and grew up in Marshalltown after his father started Wolfe Eye Clinic there. A graduate of the University of Iowa College of Medicine, Otis D. furthered his education and training in Rochester, New York, and the University of Pennsylvania.

He joined the U.S. Army Medical Corps in 1941, near the beginning of World War II. He was discharged five years later and joined his father and brother in practice at Wolfe Eye Clinic. Otis D. improved surgical procedures, invited new ideas and was a big part of why Wolfe Eye Clinic advanced throughout the 1960s and '70s. After retiring from surgery, he continued to see patients in the Marshalltown office well into his 80s. His commitment to the future of Wolfe Eye Clinic was consistently inspirational to his junior colleagues.

"He was an excellent surgeon, very, very skilled, a very competent surgeon and really enjoyed performing surgery," said Dr. John Graether, a close co-worker and friend of the Wolfe family. "Otis had carried on that innovative mindset, and I thought he was a bright guy with real good ideas."

Otis D. retired in 1991, the last of the Wolfe family to take part in the business. An accomplished photographer, many of his photos remain on display in the Marshalltown office. He died in 2006, the same year as his younger brother Russell.

RUSSELL M. WOLFE, M.D.

CATERACT EVALUATION AND SURGERY

JOINED WOLFE EYE CLINIC: 1946

LOCATION: Marshalltown

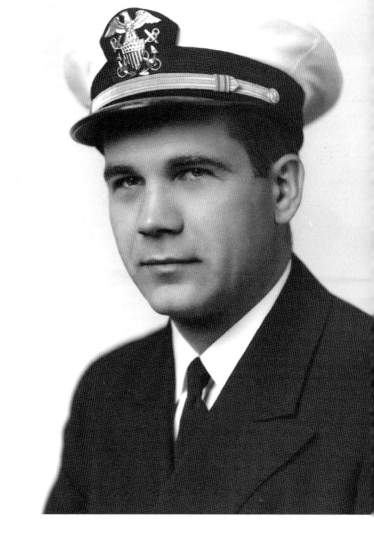

Like his father, Dr. Otis R. Wolfe, Dr. Russell Wolfe was destined to be a surgeon. He entered medical school before World War II, eventually graduating from the University of Iowa College of Medicine. He completed his medical residency in Montreal, Canada, before his years of postgraduate training at Harvard University.

Always service-oriented, Russell joined the United States Navy when America entered World War II in 1941. He was a naval flight surgeon attached to the United States. Upon his return to Marshalltown, he joined the Wolfe Eye Clinic and helped establish it as a national leader in eye care. He stayed with the clinic until 1978, when he retired to Horseshoe Bend, Arkansas, becoming an active community member.

Russell died in 2006 — he was 92 years old — and was remembered as a loyal colleague and wonderful surgeon.

"Dr. Russell excelled at his profession and was a well-known colleague to his medical peers," read an obituary in the Des Moines Sunday Register.

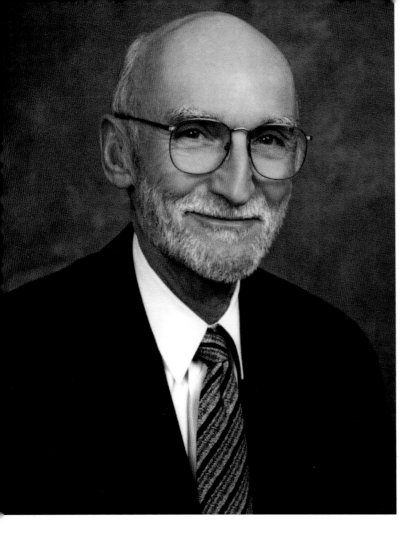

RUSSELL H. WATT, M.D.

CATARACT EVALUATION AND SURGERY

JOINED WOLFE CLINIC: 1959

LOCATION: Marshalltown

Dr. Russell Watt grew up west of Chicago in Batavia, Illinois. He did his undergraduate work at the University of Colorado and medical school at Northwestern University in Evanston, Illinois. He later completed an ophthalmology residency with the U.S. Veterans Administration and served 2 1/2 years as a U.S. Air Force flight surgeon.

"When I began looking for a position, I wanted to find a place where I would not only be fitting glasses, where there'd be enough technical support so I could work on medical eye problems," he said in an interview conducted in the late 1990s. "The Wolfes offered that, and they were very generous to us."

After joining Wolfe Eye Clinic as the first non-Wolfe family ophthalmologist, Watt was integral in the clinic's innovative and meteoric rise over the next three decades. Watt later describe the clinic as his family — he had grown up as an only child.

"As senior surgeon, Russ interviewed me in Rochester for a position at Wolfe while I was a resident at Mayo," said Dr. James Davison, the sixth eye surgeon to join Wolfe. "He was bright and warm and presented the tremendous opportunity that I might enjoy in Marshalltown. Of course, I had to follow up on that and was ultimately invited to join the practice. He loved discovering and refining new techniques and technologies. There was never a challenge too great or a detail too small. And he was right, they gave me a wonderful opportunity, the opportunity of a lifetime."

Watt performed the first corneal transplant at the clinic in 1960 and was the first, along with Dr. John Graether, in Iowa to perform phacoemulsification and intraocular lens implantation. He also did statewide outreach with fellow ophthalmologist Dr. Eric Bligard, and served as the president of the company in the late 1980s and 1990s. He retired in 1999.

JOHN M. GRAETHER, M.D.

CATARACT EVALUATION AND SURGERY

JOINED WOLFE EYE CLINIC: 1962

LOCATION: Marshalltown

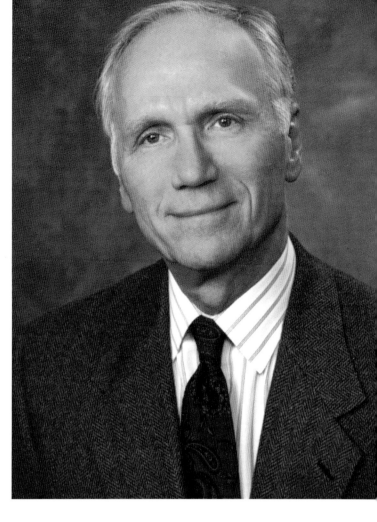

Dr. John Graether has been one of the brightest minds in the history of Wolfe Eye Clinic. Throughout his more than 50 years as a practicing ophthalmologist, Graether was granted a dozen patents, including the world's first single-piece PMMA intraocular lens, a unique device to expand the pupil during surgery, instruments for toric IOL implantation, integrated speculum eye drape, and digital and smartphone camera mounts for slit lamp photography. He continually advanced his profession through the early adoption of phacoemulsification, intraocular lens implantation and LASIK.

Graether graduated from medical school at the University of Michigan and completed his residency at the University of Iowa. Before he joined Wolfe Eye Clinic in 1962, Graether noticed a culture of innovation within the small group of physicians. It intrigued him, since he liked to try new things as well.

"The clinic already had that attitude toward accepting new ideas and innovation," said Graether, who is now retired but is actively involved in the Wolfe Foundation. "And I sensed that when I came to visit a couple of times."

Graether was the second non-Wolfe family ophthalmologist to join Wolfe Eye Clinic, and he quickly made an impact. Graether had a love for creating things, and it shined in his work. He and Dr. Watt were the first in Iowa to perform small incision phacoemulsification surgery to treat cataracts (1972) and implant intraocular lenses (1975). He independently discovered and was the first in the world to publish the perpetually significant continuous tear anterior and posterior capsulotomy procedures (capsulorhexis, 1985), and created the Graether Pupil Expander (1996), which is used around the globe today.

Graether has a love for architecture and art. He actively helped design several of the Wolfe Eye Clinic's current facilities using the same thoughtful engineering mindset assuring attractive appearance and efficient function.

Graether retired in 2013 but left behind a groundbreaking legacy. His abilities to think ahead and adopt new procedures and invent new tools are some of the biggest reasons why Wolfe Eye Clinic has earned a national reputation as an industry leader.

"I feel it's been one of my lifetime accomplishments to have been able to contribute to the clinic," Graether said. "It's still growing. And I'm very proud of the people we have acquired, and there have been a lot of them. As I've always said, 'Go out and find somebody who's smarter than you are, and don't exploit them.' That has helped us retain some of the best people out there."

Past Ophthalmologists

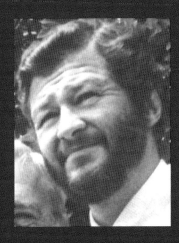

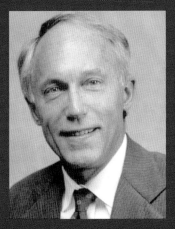

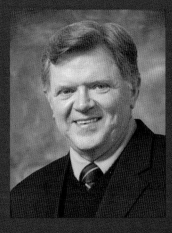

RUSSELL R. WIDNER, M.D.

SPECIALTY: Comprehensive Ophthalmology, Medical and Surgical Retina Treatment

JOINED WOLFE EYE CLINIC: 1968

LOCATION: Marshalltown

GILBERT W. HARRIS, M.D.

SPECIALTY: Cataract Evaluation and Surgery

JOINED WOLFE EYE CLINIC: 1970

LOCATION: Marshalltown

GARY L. HEDGE, M.D.

SPECIALTY: Cataract Evaluation and Surgery

JOINED WOLFE EYE CLINIC: Mid 1970s

LOCATION: Marshalltown

NORMAN F. WOODLIEF, M.D.

SPECIALTY: Retina Disease and Surgery, Cataract Evaluation and Surgery

JOINED WOLFE EYE CLINIC: 1984

LOCATIONS: Marshalltown, Cedar Falls, Cedar Rapids

EDUCATION: B.S. University of North Carolina at Greensboro, M.D.; University of North Carolina School of Medicine; Internship Mary Imogene Bassett Hospital; Residency at Wills Eye Hospital; Fellowship at Bascom Palmer Eye Institute.

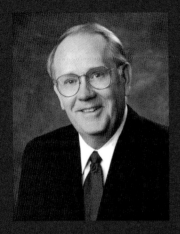

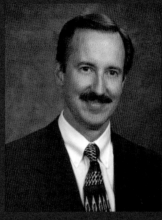

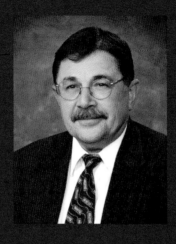

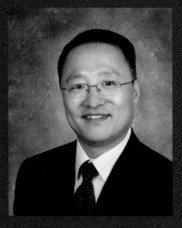

DEAN M. HARMS, M.D.

SPECIALTY: Cataract Evaluation and Surgery

JOINED WOLFE EYE CLINIC: 1997

LOCATIONS: Ames, Marshalltown

EDUCATION: B.S., Iowa State University; M.D., University of Iowa; Internship at Sacramento Medical Center; Residency at Medical College of Wisconsin.

DANIEL J. VOS, M.D.

SPECIALTY: Cataract Evaluation and Surgery

JOINED WOLFE EYE CLINIC: 1997

LOCATION: Ames

EDUCATION: B.S. University of Iowa; M.D. University of Iowa; Internship at The Marshfield Clinic & St. Joseph's Hospital; Residency at Milwaukee County Eye Institute & Affiliated Hospitals.

GREGORY A. OLSON, M.D.

SPECIALTY: Retina Disease and Surgery

JOINED WOLFE EYE CLINIC: 1997

LOCATION: Fort Dodge

EDUCATION: B.S. University of Iowa; M.D., University of Iowa; Internship at Santa Barbara County & Cottage Hospitals; Residency at Cook County Hospital.

JEONG-HYEON SOHN, M.D.

SPECIALTY: Retina Disease and Surgery

JOINED WOLFE EYE CLINIC: 2009

LOCATIONS: Cedar Rapids, Cedar Falls, Marshalltown

EDUCATION: Seoul National University; Internship at Seoul National University Hospital; Residency at Seoul National University Hospital; Fellowship at Wilmer Eye Institute.

DONNY W. SUH, M.D.

PEDIATRIC OPHTHALMOLOGY

JOINED WOLFE CLINIC: 2000

LOCATIONS: West Des Moines, Marshalltown, Ames

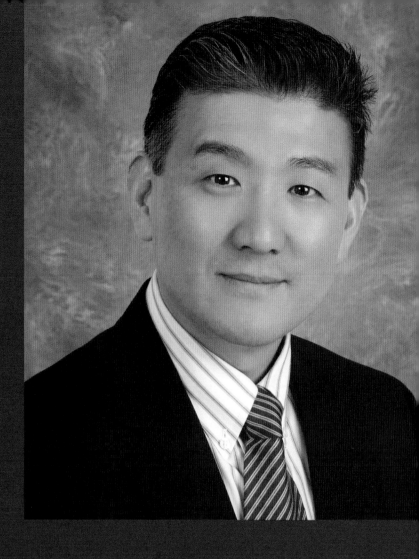

When Dr. Donny Suh was looking for a place to work after graduating from Baylor College of Medicine and finishing a fellowship at Johns Hopkins University, he was immediately attracted to Wolfe Eye Clinic. Dr. John Trible, a current physician at Wolfe Eye Clinic, was Suh's mentor during his residency. Suh also saw how the clinic treated patients.

"Their dedication to patients was second to none," Suh said. "They treated everyone with respect. It was not unusual to see some patients and staff members who had been with the clinic for 20 to 30 years."

Suh was recruited because while Wolfe Eye Clinic surgeons were successfully performing pediatric evaluations and surgery, none were formally trained pediatric ophthalmology subspecialists, and there was much more he could offer.

"I was excited about the challenge," Suh said.

Suh left Wolfe Eye Clinic to move into academics and research, but he looks back at his time fondly. He calls his 15 years with the clinic some of the "most important years of my life."

"It helped me grow. It helped me mature," Suh said. "I worked with amazing physicians who excelled in their respective fields and were mentors for me."

Ophthalmologists

JAMES A. DAVISON, M.D., FACS

CATARACT EVALUATION AND SURGERY, LASIK

JOINED WOLFE CLINIC 1980

LOCATIONS: Marshalltown, West Des Moines

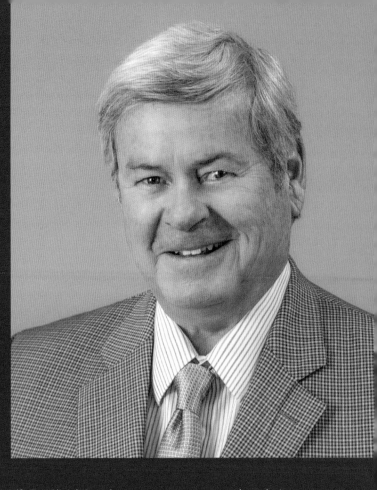

Dr. James Davison graduated summa cum laude with a bachelor's degree from the University of Minnesota. After receiving his medical degree from Mayo Medical School, Davison finished an ophthalmology internship at Los Angeles County – University of Southern California School of Medicine. He completed an ophthalmology residency at Mayo Graduate School of Medicine in Rochester, finishing as chief resident.

Following graduation, Davison had a retinal fellowship canceled at the last minute. He called one of his mentors, who connected Davison to Dr. John Graether at Wolfe Eye Clinic. Davison had never been to Marshalltown before, but he was intrigued.

"I wanted to have something that would be interesting and fun and new," Davison said. "Here are these guys in Iowa, and they were honest and nice. They were doing great science. Nobody was doing what they were doing at the time." Graether wrote to Davison that "the Wolfe Eye Clinic is about to flower," and he was certainly correct in predicting its bright future and growth.

Many credit much of Wolfe Eye Clinic's modern growth to the determination and patient care standards that Davison encompasses. As the sixth eye surgeon to join the clinic in Marshalltown, he practiced comprehensive ophthalmology performing all kinds of eye surgeries including starting the vitrectomy service. Additionally, helped grow the clinic's reach statewide and served in various leadership positions in the company, including serving as president and chairman of Wolfe Eye Clinic's Board of Directors from 1995 to 2010. Davison has continued on to serve as president of Wolfe Family Vision Centers since 1996 and Wolfe Surgery Center since 2007, and has volunteered his services to Wolfe Foundation countless times throughout his career.

Davison is a renowned surgeon, both nationally and internationally. He has performed over 70,000 cataract surgeries during his career at Wolfe Eye Clinic and successfully advanced Iowa's cataract surgery technologies by performing many "Iowa cataract surgery firsts." For example, in 2003, Davison was the first in Iowa to implant AcrySof® IQ ReSTOR® multifocal intraocular lens (IOL) as an artificial lens replacement during cataract surgery. This lens helped expand vision possibilities post-cataract surgery by reducing or eliminating the need for glasses after cataract surgery for many. In 2019, Davison was the first to implant the only FDA-approved trifocal IOL at that time, the Alcon PanOptix® Trifocal IOL.

Davison is also a highly referred to LASIK surgeon by optometrists across the Midwest and has greatly contributed to clinical ophthalmic literature, both as a writer and reviewer. Besides his many published research articles, book chapters and videos, he has served as a lecturer throughout the United States and abroad including Argentina, Canada, Chile, France, Italy, Japan and Hong Kong. He particularly enjoys instructing about cataract and LASIK surgery techniques, technology and complications management outcomes.

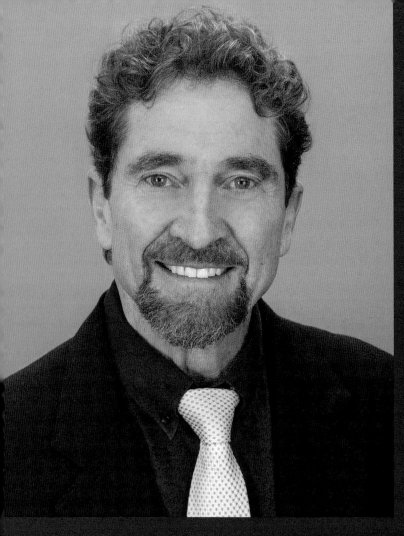

ERIC W. BLIGARD, M.D.

COMPREHENSIVE OPHTHALMOLOGY

JOINED WOLFE EYE CLINIC: 1987

LOCATION: Fort Dodge

Dr. Eric Bligard is a board-certified and fellowship-trained ophthalmologist. He received his medical degree from Johns Hopkins University and completed an ophthalmology residency and retinal fellowship at the Alton Ochsner Medical Foundation.

Dr. Bligard joined Wolfe Eye Clinic in 1987 and was the first doctor to live in a community outside of Marshalltown, working full time in the then-new Fort Dodge location. While Wolfe Eye Clinic had already opened clinics in Des Moines and Cedar Falls, the physicians were traveling there from their base in Marshalltown as the patient demand grew to the size that it would support a locally based surgeon of high caliber. Bligard grew up in a big city but moved to a small city to help grow Wolfe Eye Clinic's statewide reach.

"I initially was unwilling to consider a town or city smaller than 50,000 people," Bligard said. "However, I was persuaded that I have to look at this practice in Fort Dodge. It was described to me as a unique situation. ... I was extremely impressed."

Bligard is particularly passionate about helping those less fortunate. He has given his time, talent and resources to mission surgeries in the Philippines, Thailand, Kenya, Nicaragua, Mexico, and the People's Republic of China.

Due to a cervical neck injury leaving his right hand partially numb in 2017, Bligard is no longer operating. He has completed over 30,000 successful cataract surgeries in his career at Wolfe Eye Clinic and continues to see patients in the Fort Dodge office today. On the administrative side, Bligard was instrumental in opening outreach clinics in Emmetsburg, Algona and Estherville.

DAVID D. SAGGAU, M.D.

RETINA DISEASE AND SURGERY

JOINED WOLFE EYE CLINIC: 1990

LOCATIONS: Des Moines, Ames, Marshalltown, Pleasant Hill

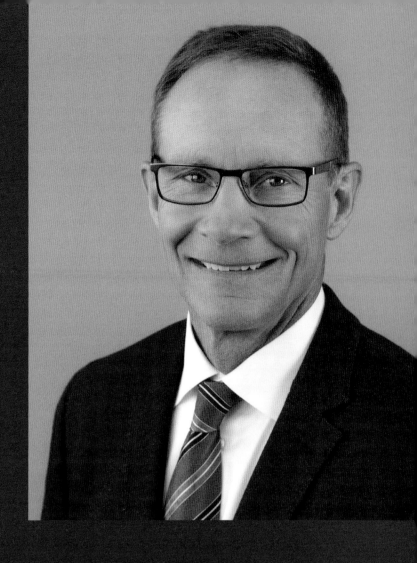

Dr. David Saggau is a board-certified and fellowship-trained retina specialist. He received his medical degree from the University of Iowa College of Medicine. Following an internship and ophthalmology residency at the Mayo Clinic, Saggau served as chief resident and assistant professor at the Illinois Eye and Ear Infirmary in Chicago. In 1990 he joined Wolfe Eye Clinic after completion of a retinal fellowship with Cleveland Retina Associates in Ohio.

At the time of his hiring in 1990, subspecialization was just beginning in ophthalmology. Saggau performed a variety of eye surgeries including cataract surgeries for five years while serving Marshalltown, Cedar Rapids, Des Moines and Fort Dodge clinics. In 1996 there was such a need for him to practice his retinal subspecialty work that he gave up all of his other surgeries. He eventually focused on retinal disease, becoming Wolfe Eye Clinic's first full-time subspecialist in retinal disease and surgery. He has led the retina team for more than two decades.

Saggau has worked tirelessly in the past 30 years to provide quality care for thousands of Iowans. He chose to become an ophthalmologist so that he could make a significant difference in his patients' quality of life. That commitment to his patients has fueled his career and sustained his energies to provide quality patient care over the past three decades.

"I would unhesitatingly pursue the same career path at the same clinic in this same great state if I could do it all over again," he said.

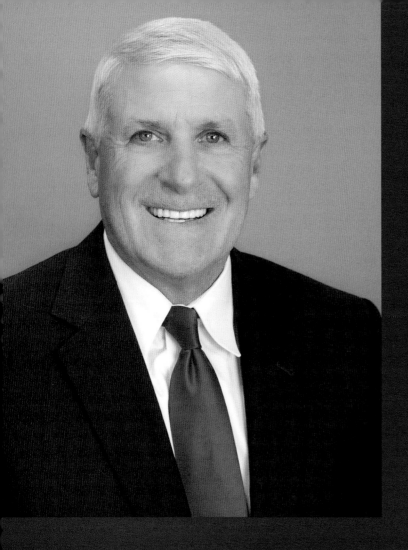

STEVEN C. JOHNSON, M.D.

CATARACT EVALUATION AND SURGERY, CORNEA DISEASE AND SURGERY, LASIK

JOINED WOLFE EYE CLINIC: 1991

LOCATION: Des Moines

Dr. Steven Johnson is a board-certified and fellowship-trained cornea transplant, LASIK and cataract specialist. After receiving his medical degree from the University of Iowa, he completed an ophthalmology residency at the University of California, San Diego, where he was chief resident. He went on to complete a corneal and anterior segment surgery fellowship at the University of Connecticut.

During the course of his fellowship in the late 1980s, Johnson worked on one of the first excimer laser prototypes used for laser vision correction surgery in the United States. He was a principal clinical investigator on the Technolas Excimer Laser and studies of LASIK laser eye surgery and PRK refractive surgery. When Johnson joined the clinic in 1991, Wolfe Eye Clinic was just getting started in its new West Des Moines office. Johnson served as the first full-time physician in the location.

In 1994 and 1995, Johnson participated in FDA trials for the excimer laser and in 1996, Johnson and his colleague, Dr. Todd Gothard, were the first ophthalmologists in Iowa to perform both PRK and LASIK eye surgery with the excimer laser. Johnson was also one of the first in central Iowa to perform intracorneal ring segment, also known as Intacs, to correct nearsightedness (myopia) in 1999. Given his extensive experience, Johnson wrote a textbook chapter on the excimer laser and astigmatism, a refractive disorder in which the cornea is irregularly shaped

He has been seeing patients with Wolfe Eye Clinic since 1991 and enjoys helping his patients meet their vision goals.

"Through my career at Wolfe Eye Clinic, we surgeons and staff have strived to practice state-of-the-art ophthalmic surgery," Johnson said.

TODD W. GOTHARD, M.D.

CORNEA DISEASE AND SURGERY, CATARACT EVALUATION AND SURGERY, LASIK

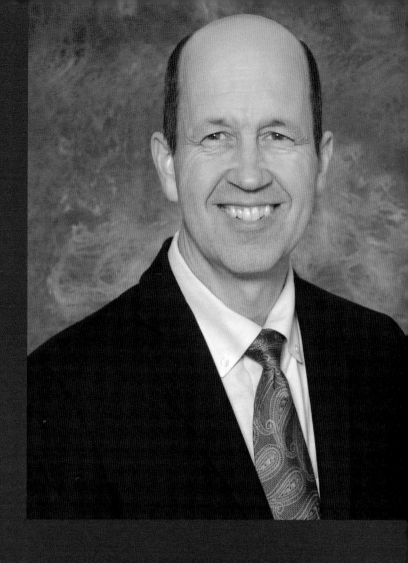

JOINED WOLFE CLINIC: 1993

LOCATIONS: Hiawatha, Iowa City

Dr. Todd Gothard is a fellowship-trained eye care specialist in refractive, corneal and cataract surgery. Gothard completed his undergraduate degree at Gannon University and earned his medical degree with honors from the University of North Carolina at Chapel Hill. Following an internship in internal medicine at the University of Pennsylvania in Philadelphia, he then completed a one-year fellowship in refractive, corneal and cataract surgery at the Phillips Eye Institute and the University of Minnesota under the direction of Dr. Richard Lindstrom.

He is an eye doctor specializing in refractive, corneal and cataract surgery and has been performing refractive surgery since 1990. He joined Wolfe Eye Clinic in 1993 and was the first full-time physician placed in the Cedar Rapids office. Gothard enjoys seeing the reactions of his patients, particularly when they come in after a life-changing surgery.

Over the years, Gothard has been actively involved in clinical trials, including one for the excimer laser in 1994. After participation in the FDA trials, Gothard and his colleague, Dr. Steven Johnson, were the first ophthalmologists in Iowa to perform both PRK and LASIK eye surgery with the excimer laser. Gothard was also one of the first in central Iowa to perform intracorneal ring segment, also known as Intacs, to correct nearsightedness (myopia) in 1999.

"I really enjoy helping people to see better, both with their glasses or without their glasses," Gothard said. "It's always very fun to come in the day after people have had LASIK surgery and see the smiles on their faces just because they can see things they haven't been able to see before."

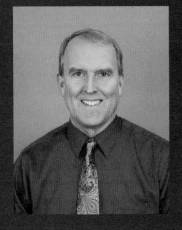

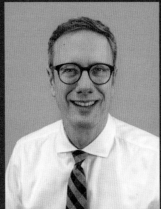

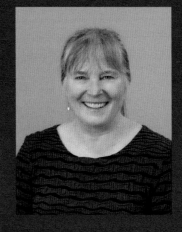

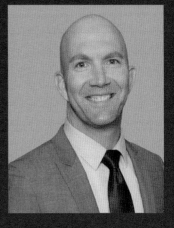

LOUIS J. SCALLON, M.D.

SPECIALTY: Cataract Evaluation and Surgery, Comprehensive Ophthalmology, LASIK

JOINED WOLFE EYE CLINIC: 1997

LOCATION: Ames

EDUCATION: M.D., University of Iowa College Medicine; Residency at Medical College of Wisconsin, Milwaukee Country Medical Complex.

CHARLES H. BARNES, M.D.

SPECIALTY: Retinal Disease and Surgery

JOINED WOLFE EYE CLINIC: 1997

LOCATIONS: Hiawatha, Cedar Falls, Waterloo

EDUCATION: B.S., Graceland College; M.D., University of Iowa College of Medicine; Internship at Broadlawns Medical Center; Residency at Texas Tech University Health and Science Center; Fellowship at University of Nebraska Medical Center (retinal medicine and surgery).

LEANN J. LARSON, M.D.

SPECIALTY: Comprehensive Ophthalmology

JOINED WOLFE EYE CLINIC: 1999

LOCATIONS: Hiawatha, Iowa City

EDUCATION: B.S., St. Olaf University; M.D., Washington University; Residency at Washington University.

BENJAMIN L. MASON, M.D.

SPECIALTY: Cataract Evaluation and Surgery, Glaucoma, LASIK

JOINED WOLFE EYE CLINIC: 2006

LOCATIONS: Cedar Falls, Waterloo

EDUCATION: B.S., University of Iowa; M.D., University of Iowa College of Medicine; Residency and Fellowship at Bascom Palmer Eye Institute (glaucoma).

JOHN R. TRIBLE, M.D.

CATARACT EVALUATION AND SURGERY, GLAUCOMA

JOINED WOLFE CLINIC 1998

LOCATIONS: Des Moines, Marshalltown

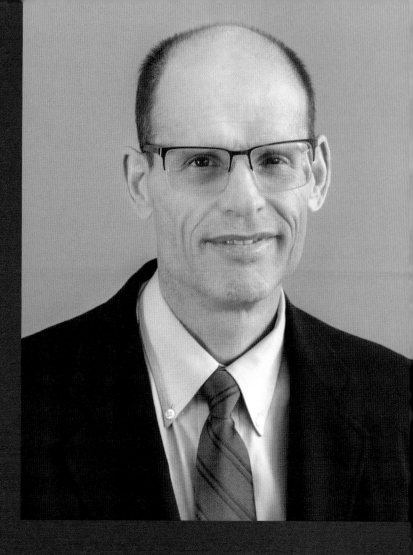

Dr. John Trible is a board-certified and fellowship-trained glaucoma specialist who has been helping patients with Wolfe Eye Clinic since 1998. He received his medical degree from Georgetown University School of Medicine. Following an ophthalmology residency at Wills Eye Hospital, Trible completed a glaucoma fellowship at Bascom Palmer Eye Institute. Before joining Wolfe Eye Clinic, Trible served on the ophthalmology teaching and research staff at the Eye Institute of the Medical College of Wisconsin.

Trible was the first full-time glaucoma subspecialist to join the Wolfe Eye Clinic staff. He was one of the first to do a tube shunt procedure, called an Aqueous Drainage Device, and later performed the first selective laser trabeculoplasty (SLT) procedure at Wolfe Eye Clinic, further expanding Wolfe Eye Clinic's glaucoma treatment options and improving outcomes for many glaucoma patients. Trible also contributed greatly to the field in 2007, when he was the first in Iowa to begin performing glaucoma surgery with the use of a Trabectome, which is a surgical devise that makes glaucoma surgery less invasive. He has published many scientific papers, contributed a chapter to the second edition of the Wills Eye Manual and lectured widely on topics within his specialty.

Trible enjoys the complex, problem-solving nature of ophthalmology as well as the opportunity to help people and make an impact in his patients' lives.

"I enjoy taking care of our glaucoma patients," Trible said. "I feel people really need the help, and patients are really enjoyable to work with."

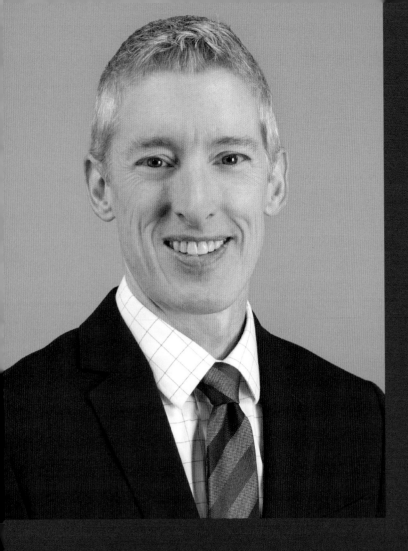

DOUGLAS R. CASADY, M.D

OCULOFACIAL PLASTICS

JOINED WOLFE CLINIC: 2005

LOCATIONS: Des Moines, Ames, Fort Dodge, Marshalltown

Dr. Douglas Casady was the first oculoplastic surgeon to join Wolfe Eye Clinic, more than a decade ago. Before joining the clinic, Casady completed a fellowship at the Lions Eye Institute in Albany, New York, where he received the Golden Apple teaching award from the residents at Albany Medical College. Prior to his fellowship, he completed his residency at Scott & White Memorial Hospital, Texas A&M University College of Medicine, where he was chief resident. He graduated from the Creighton University School of Medicine.

Since he was one of the few oculoplastic surgeons in Iowa, Casady traveled all over the state in his first few years with the clinic. He has also traveled to the Dominican Republic multiple times to provide medical and surgical care.

JARED S. NIELSEN, M.D, M.B.A.

RETINA DISEASE AND SURGERY, DIRECTOR OF CLINICAL TRIALS

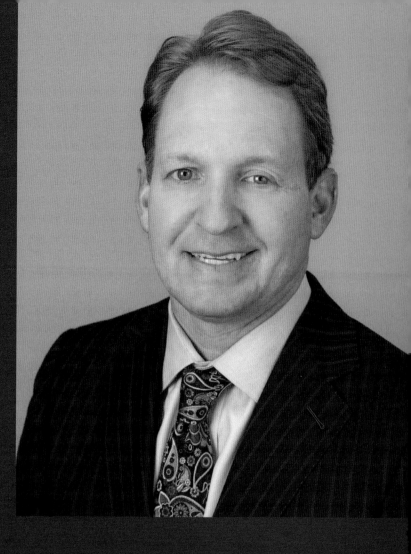

JOINED WOLFE CLINIC: 2007

LOCATIONS: Des Moines, Ames, Fort Dodge, Pleasant Hill

Dr. Jared Nielsen earned his medical degree along with a master's degree in pathology in a combined degree program at the Chicago Medical School. Following a transitional internship at the University of Hawaii, he completed an ophthalmology residency at Loyola University Chicago. Nielsen completed a vitreoretinal surgery fellowship at Northwestern University, where he remains a clinical instructor of ophthalmology.

Nielsen has been integral in building up the organization's active participation in medical research, which was a driving force in his decision to join Wolfe Eye Clinic more than a decade ago.

"One of the reasons I came to the clinic was because it's a leader in eye care," Nielsen said.

He has served as a principal investigator in nearly 50 clinical trials advancing care for patients who suffer from blinding diseases including wet and dry macular degeneration, diabetic retinopathy and central serous chorioretinopathy. He is engaged as an investigator in the DRCR Retina Network, a National Eye Institute-sponsored effort to study retinal disease.

Nielsen got into ophthalmology because he could see the difference he was making in patients' lives.

"As I did my rotations in medical school, I saw that when you can provide something to help with someone's vision, you can really change their life," Nielsen said. "I'm really grateful for the opportunity that ophthalmology has to help other people and improve people's lives."

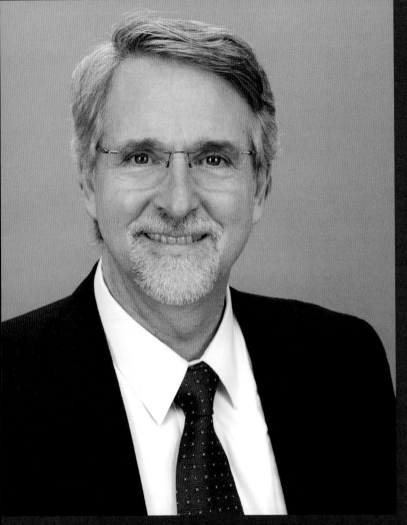

STEPHEN A. FOX, M.D.

CATARACT EVALUATION AND SURGERY, COMPREHENSIVE OPHTHALMOLOGY

JOINED WOLFE CLINIC: 2008

LOCATION: Spencer

Dr. Stephen Fox has always been passionate about helping others. From the moment he joined Wolfe Eye Clinic in 2008 to serve the Fort Dodge location, he has always provided a higher standard of care for the communities and patients he serves. Within a few years of joining the clinic, Fox was integral in opening the Spencer location in 2011.

He realized ophthalmology was the field for him when he learned about 20 million people are blinded across the world due to cataracts. That's why he participates in global mission trips in countries such as Guatemala and Ecuador, performing cataract surgery and training other ophthalmologists in manual small incision cataract surgery.

"This is a needed service," Fox said. "There are 20 million people in the world that are blind in both eyes, and they don't have any one to give them care. This looked like a field where I could make a difference. And it looked like a field where I could live in a small city and provide service. That was always my dream."

Fox earned his doctorate of medicine from the Indiana University School of Medicine. Following an internship at St. Vincent Hospital Health Care Associates, Fox completed an ophthalmology residency at the University of Michigan Medical Center.

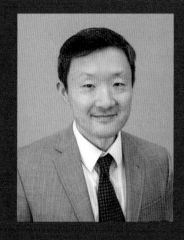

PETER RHEE, M.D.

SPECIALTY: Cataract Evaluation and Surgery, Comprehensive Ophthalmology

JOINED WOLFE EYE CLINIC: 2008

LOCATIONS: Cedar Falls, Marshalltown, Waterloo

EDUCATION: B.A., University of Chicago; M.D., The John Hopkins University School of Medicine; Internship at The Mary Imogene Bassett Hospital; Residency at The Eye Institute, Medical College of Wisconsin, Madison.

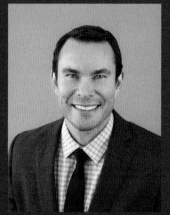

KYLE J. ALLIMAN, M.D.

SPECIALTY: Retina Disease and Surgery

JOINED WOLFE EYE CLINIC: 2010

LOCATIONS: Des Moines, Ames, Fort Dodge, Ottumwa

EDUCATION: B.S., University of Northern Iowa; M.D., University of Iowa College of Medicine; Internship, Iowa Methodist Hospital; Residency and Fellowship at Bascom Palmer Eye Institute (vitreoretinal surgery).

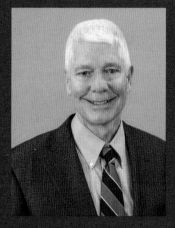

GREGORY L. THORGAARD, M.D.

SPECIALTY: Comprehensive Ophthalmology

JOINED WOLFE EYE CLINIC: 2014

LOCATION: Ottumwa

EDUCATION: B.S., Arizona State University; M.D., University of Iowa College of Medicine; Residency at University of Iowa College of Medicine.

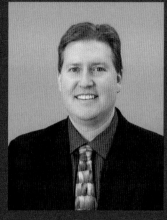

RYAN D. VINCENT, M.D.

SPECIALTY: Cataract Evaluation and Surgery, Glaucoma

JOINED WOLFE EYE CLINIC: 2014

LOCATIONS: Ottumwa, Ames, Pleasant Hill, Des Moines, Marshalltown

EDUCATION: B.S., Colorado State University; M.D., University of Colorado and Health Sciences Center School of Medicine; Residency at University of Missouri – Kansas City, School of Medicine; Fellowship at Baylor College of Medicine (glaucoma).

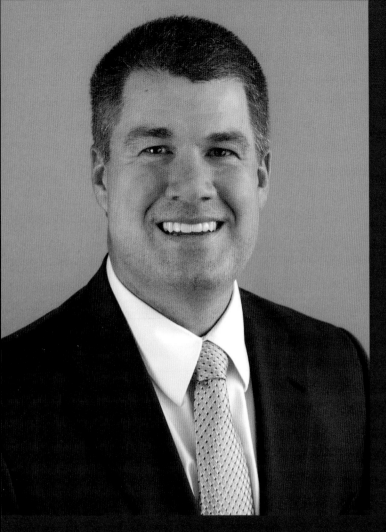

MATTHEW P. RAUEN, M.D.

CORNEA DISEASE AND SURGERY, CATARACT EVALUATION AND SURGERY, LASIK

JOINED WOLFE CLINIC: 2002

LOCATIONS: West Des Moines, Fort Dodge

Dr. Matthew Rauen earned his medical degree from the University of Iowa, where he also completed his ophthalmology residency followed by a cornea, external disease and refractive surgery fellowship. Rauen was recognized during his time at the University of Iowa for his teaching efforts with medical student and resident teaching

As a corneal specialist, Rauen's clinical practice is devoted to the front portion of the eye. His refractive cataract practice incorporates the newest possible technologies to offer patients additional spectacle independence after surgery, and his cornea practice is devoted to the newest forms of corneal transplantation. Rauen was the first Wolfe Eye Clinic surgeon

Keratoplasty) and in 2016, Rauen was the first surgeon in central Iowa to perform collagen cross linking with the KXL® System — a corneal treatment that has become the gold standard for treating progressive keratoconus.

For patients who may be better suited for refractive procedures other than LASIK, Rauen

Refractive Lens Exchange (RLE). He was the first surgeon in Iowa to implant a toric ICL in 2019, expanding vision correction options for patients with astigmatism.

Above all, Rauen does not believe in a "one-size-fits-all" approach. He enjoys patient education and believes this better allows care decisions.

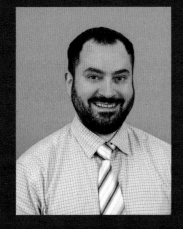 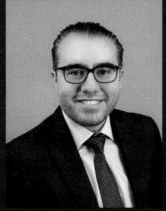 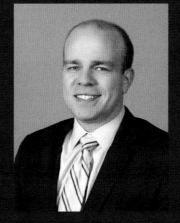 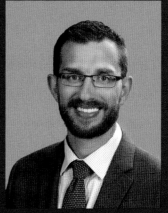

ALEX KARTVELISHVILI, M.D.

SPECIALTY: Retina Disease and Surgery

JOINED WOLFE EYE CLINIC: 2015

LOCATIONS: Iowa City, Cedar Falls, Hiawatha, Marshalltown, Ottumwa

EDUCATION: B.S., Hunter College at the State University of

GEORGE J. PAR, M.D.

SPECIALTY: Retina Disease and Surgery

JOINED WOLFE EYE CLINIC: 2016

LOCATIONS: Des Moines, Ottumwa

EDUCATION: B.A., New York University; M.D., New York University School of Medicine; Residency at New

DEREK P. BITNER, M.D.

SPECIALTY: Pediatric Ophthalmology, Strabismus

JOINED WOLFE EYE CLINIC: 2016

LOCATIONS: Des Moines, Marshalltown

EDUCATION: B.S., University of Arizona; M.D., Baylor College of Medicine; Residency at Dean McGee Eye Institute/University

PAUL S. BOEKE, M.D.

SPECIALTY: Retina Disease and Surgery

JOINED WOLFE EYE CLINIC: 2017

LOCATIONS: Cedar Falls, Hiawatha, Iowa City, Marshalltown, Waterloo

EDUCATION: B.S., University of Iowa; M.D., University of Iowa College of Medicine; Internship

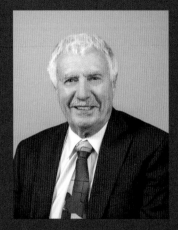

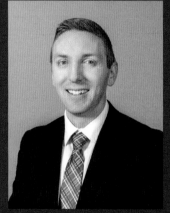

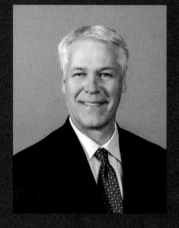

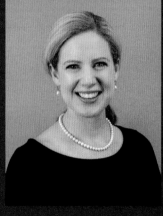

GEORGE B. CLAVENNA, D.O.

SPECIALTY: Comprehensive Ophthalmology

JOINED WOLFE EYE CLINIC: 2018

LOCATIONS: Des Moines, Pleasant Hill

EDUCATION: B.S. and M.S., Wayne State University; M.P.H.

REID P. TURNER, M.D.

SPECIALTY: Cataract Evaluation and Surgery, Corneal Disease, LASIK

JOINED WOLFE EYE CLINIC: 2018

LOCATIONS: Des Moines, Marshalltown, Ottumwa, Pleasant Hill

EDUCATION: B.A., Central

STEVEN O. ANDERSON, M.D.

SPECIALTY: Cataract Evaluation and Surgery, Comprehensive Ophthalmology

JOINED WOLFE EYE CLINIC: 2018

LOCATIONS: Ames, Fort Dodge, Marshalltown

EDUCATION: B.S.,

ANNE M. LANGGUTH, M.D.

SPECIALTY: Pediatric Ophthalmology, Strabismus

JOINED WOLFE EYE CLINIC: 2019

LOCATIONS: Hiawatha, Iowa City, Waterloo

EDUCATION: B.A., Harvard University; M.D.,

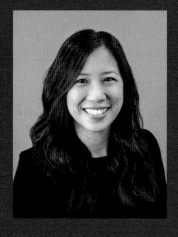 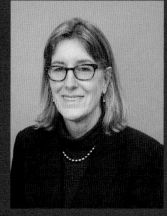

AUDREY C. KO, M.D.

SPECIALTY: Oculofacial Plastics

JOINED WOLFE EYE CLINIC: 2019

LOCATIONS: Des Moines, Ames, Cedar Falls, Fort Dodge, Marshalltown, Ottumwa

EDUCATION: B.S., University of Arizona; M.D., University of Iowa College of Medicine; Residency at Bascom Palmer Eye Institute; Fellowship at Shiley Eye Institute at University of California – San Diego (ASOPRS accredited oculoplastics).

JEAN B. SPENCER, M.D.

SPECIALTY: Pediatric Ophthalmology, Strabismus

JOINED WOLFE EYE CLINIC: 2019

LOCATION: West Des Moines

EDUCATION: B.S., Iowa State University; M.D., University of Iowa Hospitals and Clinics; Residency at University of Iowa Hospitals and Clinics; Fellowship at University of Chicago and Children's Memorial Hospital (pediatric ophthalmology).

Past

Optometrists

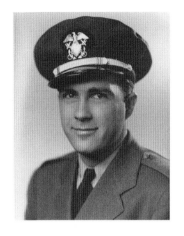

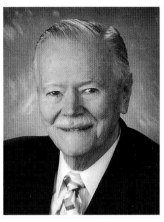

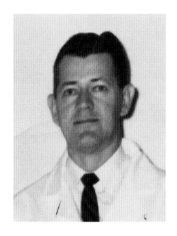

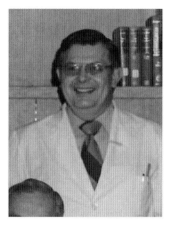

HENRY L. WOLFE, O.D.

SPECIALTY: Optometry

JOINED WOLFE EYE CLINIC: 1945

LOCATION: Marshalltown

HARRY RASDAHL, O.D.

SPECIALTY: Optometry

JOINED WOLFE EYE CLINIC: 1955

LOCATION: Marshalltown

JERRY P. NESSET, O.D.

SPECIALTY: Optometry

JOINED WOLFE EYE CLINIC: 1949

LOCATION: Marshalltown

EDUCATION: B.S. University of California-Berkeley; O.D. Northern Illinois College of Optometry

DORAL T. CHAPMAN, O.D.

SPECIALTY: Optometry

JOINED WOLFE EYE CLINIC: Mid 1950s

LOCATION: Marshalltown

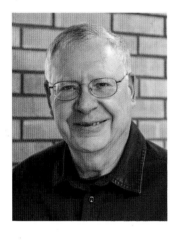

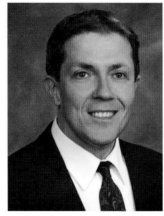

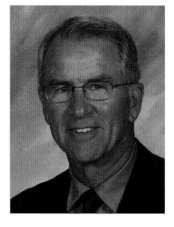

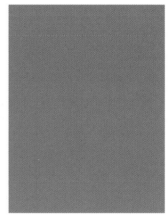

PETE R. STERZING, O.D.

SPECIALTY: Optometry

JOINED WOLFE EYE CLINIC: 1974

LOCATION: Marshalltown

JOSEPH W. JOHLL, O.D.

SPECIALTY: Optometry

JOINED WOLFE EYE CLINIC: 1996

LOCATION: Fairfield

EDUCATION: B.S., Viterbo College; O.D., Illinois College of Optometry.

ROBERT J. NIEMAN, O.D.

SPECIALTY: Optometry

JOINED WOLFE EYE CLINIC: 1998

LOCATION: Webster City

EDUCATION: B.A., Wartburg College; O.D., Illinois College of Optometry.

DANIELLE FEE, O.D.

SPECIALTY: Optometry

JOINED WOLFE EYE CLINIC: 1998

LOCATION: Marshalltown

EDUCATION: B.A., Simpson College; O.D., Michigan College of Optometry. BA Simpson College, medical: Michigan College of Optometry

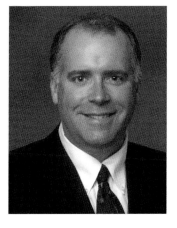

TODD A. VERDON, O.D.

SPECIALTY: Optometry

JOINED WOLFE EYE CLINIC: 1998

LOCATIONS: Waverly, Marshalltown

EDUCATION: B.A., University of Northern Iowa; O.D., Illinois College of Optometry.

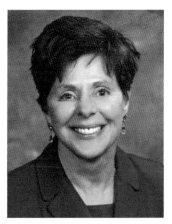

PATRICIA A. BLUME, O.D.

SPECIALTY: Optometry

JOINED WOLFE CLINIC: 1999

LOCATION: Fairfield

EDUCATION: B.A. and O.D., University of Missouri.

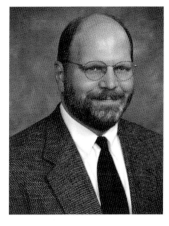

MARSHALL K. WALKER, O.D.

SPECIALTY: Optometry

JOINED WOLFE EYE CLINIC: 1999

LOCATION: Tama

EDUCATION: B.A., Northern Michigan University and University of Oklahoma; O.D., Illinois College of Optometry.

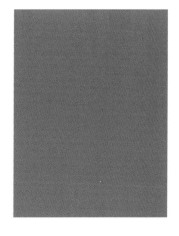

JERRY GIBSON, O.D.

SPECIALTY: Optometry

JOINED WOLFE EYE CLINIC: 2004

LOCATIONS: Fairfield, Sigourney

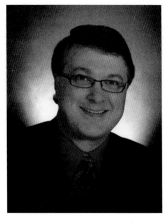

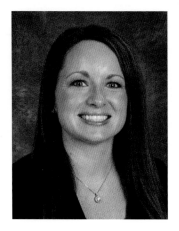

KREG D. HARPER, O.D

SPECIALTY: Optometry

JOINED WOLFE EYE CLINIC: 2008

LOCATIONS: Fairfield, Sigourney, Keokuk

EDUCATION: B.A., University of Northern Iowa; O.D., Illinois College of Optometry; Fellowship Illinois at Minnesota Eye Consultants

SARAH A. SLIWINSKI, O.D.

SPECIALTY: Optometry

JOINED WOLFE EYE CLINIC: 2014

LOCATION: Fairfield

EDUCATION: B.A., Wartburg College; O.D. Illinois College of Optometry.

Optometrists

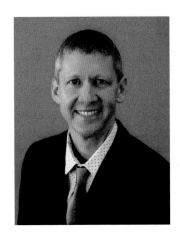

JAMES. C. TESDAHL, O.D.

SPECIALTY: Optometry

JOINED WOLFE FAMILY VISION CENTER: 1998

LOCATION: Webster City

EDUCATION: B.A., Coe College; O.D., Indiana School of Optometry.

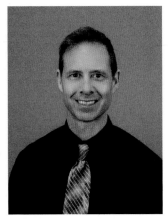

CORY L. BOWER, O.D

SPECIALTY: Optometry

JOINED WOLFE EYE CLINIC: 1999

LOCATIONS: Hiawatha, Marshalltown

EDUCATION: B.A., Simpson College; O.D., Illinois College of Optometry.

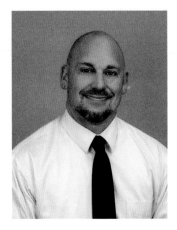

CHAD A. GIDEL, O.D.

SPECIALTY: Optometry

JOINED WOLFE EYE CLINIC: 1999

LOCATION: Ames

EDUCATION: B.A., University of Illinois and St. Crois State University; O.D., Illinois College of Optometry.

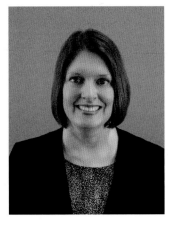

DENISE C. GIMBEL, O.D.

SPECIALTY: Optometry

JOINED WOLFE EYE CLINIC: 2000

LOCATION: Marshalltown

EDUCATION: B.A., Central College; O.D., Illinois College of Optometry; Residency at Tuscaloosa Veterans Administration Medical Center.

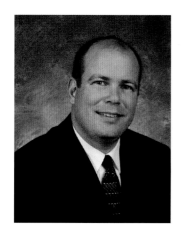

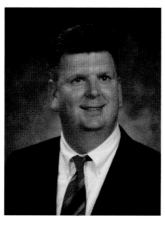

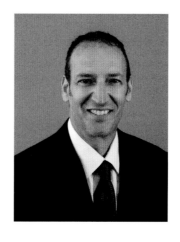

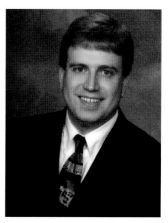

JOHN P. FERRELL, O.D.

SPECIALTY: Optometry

JOINED WOLFE FAMILY VISION CENTER: 2000

LOCATION: Webster City

EDUCATION: B.A., Wartburg College; O.D., Illinois College of Optometry.

THOMAS R. MUNGER, O.D.

SPECIALTY: Optometry

JOINED WOLFE FAMILY VISION CENTER: 2002

LOCATION: Sac City

EDUCATION: B.S., Dana College; O.D., Southern College of Optometry; Residency at Family Practice Optometry West Tennessee Eye.

MARK G. HOLMES, O.D.

SPECIALTY: Optometry

JOINED WOLFE EYE CLINIC: 2003

LOCATION: Des Moines

EDUCATION: B.S., Iowa State University; O.D., Indiana School of Optometry.

MARK H. JEPPESEN, O.D.

SPECIALTY: Optometry

JOINED WOLFE FAMILY VISION CENTER: 2003

LOCATION: Waverly

EDUCATION: B.A., Concordia College – Moorehead, Minnesota; O.D., Illinois College of Optometry.

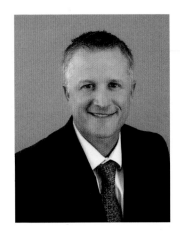

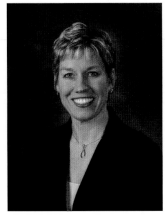

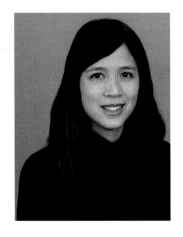

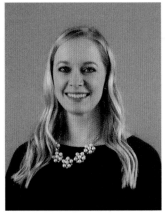

JUSTIN M. SCHULTE, O.D.

SPECIALTY: Optometry

JOINED WOLFE EYE CLINIC: 2003

LOCATION: Des Moines

EDUCATION: B.A., Central College; O.D., Illinois College of Optometry.

CHRISTINE L. SEMLER-BLUE, O.D.

SPECIALTY: Optometry

JOINED WOLFE FAMILY VISION CENTER: 2004

LOCATION: Story City

EDUCATION: B.A., Central College; O.D., Pacific University College of Optometry.

MYRA N. MENDOZA, O.D.

SPECIALTY: Optometry, Pediatric Optometry

JOINED WOLFE EYE CLINIC: 2008

LOCATIONS: Des Moines, Ames, Marshalltown

EDUCATION: B.S. and O.D., University of California at Berkeley.

SARA D. KHAN, O.D.

SPECIALTY: Optometry, Pediatric Optometry

JOINED WOLFE EYE CLINIC: 2012

LOCATION: Des Moines

EDUCATION: B.A., University of Iowa; O.D., Southern College of Optometry.

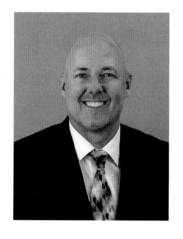

JEFFREY P. COLLETT, O.D.

SPECIALTY: Optometry

JOINED WOLFE EYE CLINIC: 2014

LOCATION: Ottumwa

EDUCATION: B.A., University of Iowa; O.D., Southern College of Optometry.

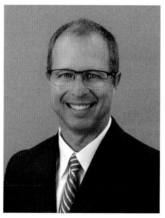

R. PAYSON MORELAND, O.D.

SPECIALTY: Optometry

JOINED WOLFE EYE CLINIC: 2014

LOCATIONS: Ottumwa, Albia

EDUCATION: B.S., Central College; O.D., University of Missouri – St. Louis; Residency at John Cochran Veteran's Hospital (ocular disease).

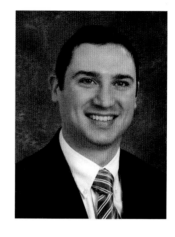

DANIEL R. SLIWINSKI, O.D.

SPECIALTY: Optometry

JOINED WOLFE FAMILY VISION CENTER: 2014

LOCATIONS: Fairfield, Sigourney, Keokuk

EDUCATION: B.A., Marquette University; O.D., Illinois College of Optometry.

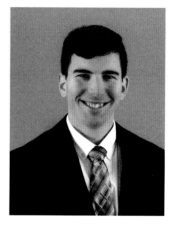

KEATON C. CORNISH, O.D

SPECIALTY: Optometry

JOINED WOLFE EYE CLINIC: 2014

LOCATIONS: Des Moines, Marshalltown

EDUCATION: B.A, University of Northern Iowa; O.D., Illinois College of Optometry; Residency at Kansas City Veterans Administration Medical Center.

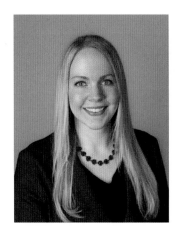

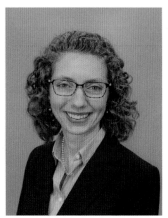

SARA R. PATIN, O.D.

SPECIALTY: Optometry

JOINED WOLFE FAMILY VISION CENTER: 2015

LOCATIONS: Toledo, Traer

EDUCATION: B.A., Augustana College; O.D., Illinois College of Optometry.

SARA. E. OLSON, O.D.

SPECIALTY: Optometry, Pediatric Optometry

JOINED WOLFE EYE CLINIC: 2019

LOCATION: Des Moines

EDUCATION: B.S., Minnesota State University, O.D., Pacific University College of Optometry.

Past Ear, Nose, Throat

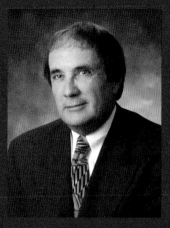 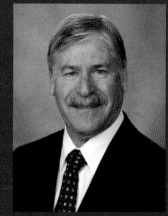

MICHAEL W. HILL, M.D.

SPECIALTY: Ears, Nose and Throat

JOINED WOLFE EYE CLINIC: 1977

LOCATIONS: Marshalltown, Des Moines

EDUCATION: University of Iowa College of Medicine; Internship at Santa Clara Valley Medical Center; Residency at Stanford University (specialty training in head and neck surgery and facial plastic and reconstructive surgery).

DANIEL J. BLUM, M.D.

SPECIALTY: Ears, Nose and Throat

JOINED WOLFE EYE CLINIC: 1984

LOCATION: Marshalltown, Cedar Falls

EDUCATION: Creighton University School of Medicine; Residency at Mayo Clinic College of Medicine and Science.

Past Audiologists

BRUCE E. VIRCKS, AU. D.

AUDIOLOGY

JOINED WOLFE AUDIOLOGY: 1983

LOCATIONS: Ames, Cedar Falls, Marshalltown, West Des Moines

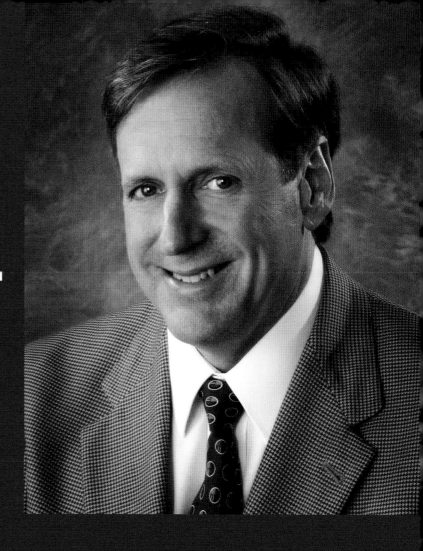

Dr. Bruce Vircks joined Wolfe Eye Clinic in 1983 as its first audiologist. Based in Marshalltown, he later became the driving force behind the creation of an Audiology Department within the Clinic. As director, he oversaw the growth of the department into four locations (Ames, Marshalltown, Cedar Falls and West Des Moines), performing both diagnostic and dispensing practices. Before retiring in 2018, he specialized in audiology, hearing conservation, hearing aids and Lyric extended-wear instruments.

Throughout his career, Vircks focused on hearing conservation programs to reduce noise exposure, as well as hearing aid technology, including extended-wear instruments. Vircks was active in both state and national audiology organizations and enjoyed presenting information to fellow audiologists on hearing conservation, audiology practice models, cerumen management and hearing aid technology. In 2011, he was elected president of the Academy of Doctors of Audiology, an organization dedicated to the advancement of practitioner excellence and quality audiologic care.

Vircks attended University of Wisconsin-Madison where he received his master's in audiology, and later received a doctorate in audiology from the Arizona School of Health Sciences.

  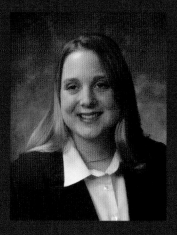

DEB S. RIEKS, AU. D.

SPECIALTY: Audiology

JOINED WOLFE AUDIOLOGY: 1992

LOCATION: Cedar Falls

EDUCATION: B.A. and M.A., University of Northern Iowa; Au. D., Arizona School of Health Sciences.

SARAH HAWKER, AU. D.

SPECIALTY: Audiology

JOINED WOLFE AUDIOLOGY: 1998

LOCATION: Cedar Falls

EDUCATION: B.A., University of Northern Iowa; M.A. and Aud. D., University of Iowa.

JESSICA WILLIAMS, AU. D.

SPECIALTY: Audiology

JOINED WOLFE AUDIOLOGY: 2000

LOCATION: Marshalltown

EDUCATION: B.A. and M.A., University of Northern Iowa.

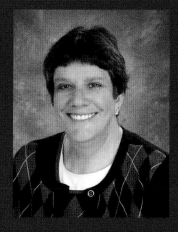 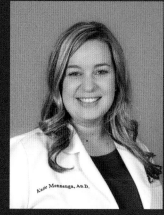

CATHERINE M. DANGELSER, AU. D.

SPECIALTY: Audiology

JOINED WOLFE AUDIOLOGY: 2004

LOCATIONS: Marshalltown, Ames

EDUCATION: B.S., University of Wisconsin-Stevens Point; M.A., Western Michigan University; Au. D., University of Florida Gainesville.

KATIE E. MENNENGA, AU. D.

SPECIALTY: Audiology

JOINED WOLFE AUDIOLOGY: 2004

LOCATION: Cedar Falls

EDUCATION: Au. D., Northern Illinois University.

Audiologists

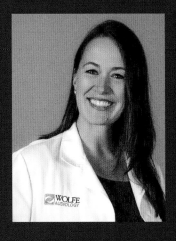 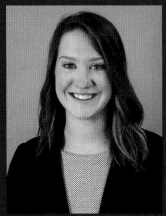

ROBYN L. RITCHEY, AU. D.

SPECIALTY: Audiology

JOINED WOLFE AUDIOLOGY: 2016

LOCATION: Marshalltown

EDUCATION: B.A. and M.S., University of Northern Iowa; Au. D., Arizona School of Health Scientists

CHRISTINE E. MCGUINTY, AU. D., CCC-A

SPECIALTY: Audiology

JOINED WOLFE AUDIOLOGY: 2019

LOCATIONS: Marshalltown, Cedar Falls

EDUCATION: B.A., University of Northern Iowa; Au. Do, University of Wisconsin – Madison.

Fellowship Program

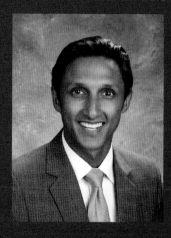 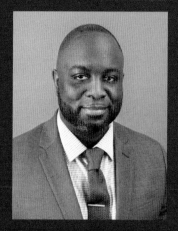

2019 Graduate	**2021 Graduate**

DEEPAK MANGLA, M.D.

SPECIALTY: Vitreoretinal Fellow

JOINED WOLFE EYE CLINIC: 2017

LOCATIONS: West Des Moines

EDUCATION: M.D., Albany Medical College; Residency at McGaw Medical Center of Northwestern University; Fellowship at Wolfe Eye Clinic (vitreoretinal).

IAN THOMPSON, M.D.

SPECIALTY: Vitreoretinal Fellow

JOINED WOLFE EYE CLINIC: 2019

LOCATIONS: West Des Moines

EDUCATION: Harvard University; M.D., Case Western Reserve School of Medicine; Residency at Vanderbilt University Medical School; Fellowship Uveitis and Ocular Immunology, NEI/NIH.

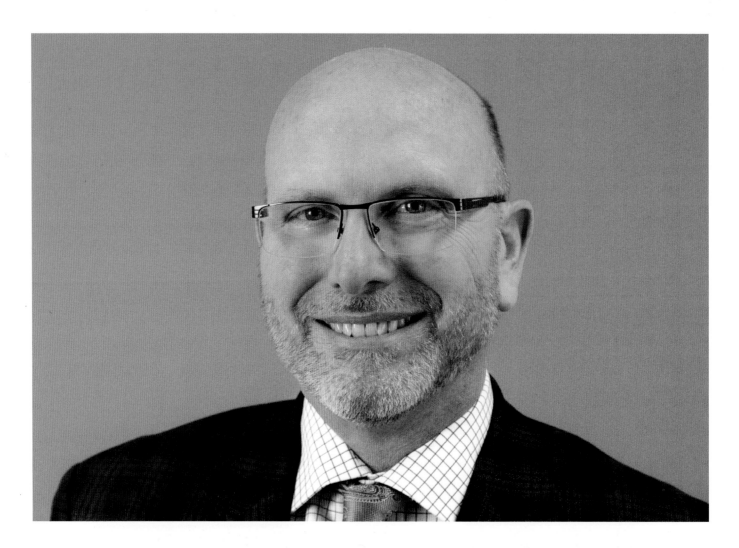

KEVIN SWARTZ
A Leader Behind Success

Kevin Swartz likes to joke that he didn't exactly know the difference between ophthalmology and optometry when he first joined Wolfe Eye Clinic as its chief executive officer in 1993. But Swartz had the personality, and he certainly had the business know-how, that has since translated to consistent success.

More than 25 years later, Wolfe Eye Clinic has expanded across Iowa and is enjoying some of its best years under Swartz's leadership, even if there was an initial learning curve.

"I think day one I learned the difference between an optometrist and an ophthalmologist," Swartz said with a laugh. "I've had a great team to help me. My role as a CEO is to help guide the Board of Directors, which is made up of physician owners. It's always been a cooperative environment where we work together and make decisions based off each other's input."

Swartz didn't have formal health care experience, but his business knowledge was vast. An Iowa native, Swartz grew up on a farm near Dolliver, Iowa, and attended the University of Northern Iowa. He had held several positions in public accounting early in his career, taking a variety of leadership and consulting roles, being a recruiter and a CFO of a startup horse racing facility, Prairie Meadows, before joining Wolfe Eye Clinic and moving to Marshalltown in 1993.

At first, Swartz was sent to Wolfe Eye Clinic by an accounting firm on an interim basis. The business was reeling from a systematic embezzlement by a previous administrator, and it was up to Swartz to right the ship. Swartz impressed the Wolfe physicians, and several months later he was asked to stay on permanently.

"Twenty-seven years later we continue to realize that we made a wonderful choice," said Dr. James Davison, a Wolfe surgeon since 1980. "He was a really bright guy, very intuitive, loving and caring, optimistic and hardworking, generous and honest and had that all-important great sense of humor."

The mid-1990s were one of the busiest and exhilarating times in Wolfe Eye Clinic history. New locations were opening across the state, and satellite offices were expanding the clinic's reach into rural communities. It would seem Swartz had his work cut out for him.

"Kevin has had a tremendous impact on the clinic," said Dr. John Graether, who joined Wolfe Eye Clinic in 1962 and was a physician owner for more than 50 years. "Kevin has kept an especially good leadership core. In my career, management became increasingly important, particularly as our practice began to expand. Without good management, we never would have succeeded."

Davison added: "He turned our small group practice into a large, sophisticated organization."

Under Swartz's leadership, the business followed the lead of physicians. Innovation and new ideas were keys in advancing Wolfe Eye Clinic's business model and structure. When he began, Swartz gathered his team and went through a strategic planning process. Part of that was creating mission and vision statements. Swartz helped chart the path forward.

In 1997, Swartz spearheaded the merger with another ophthalmology practice in central Iowa. At the time, Wolfe Eye Clinic had 125 employees and 12 medical doctors serving five locations in Iowa. Fast-forward to 2019 and Wolfe Eye Clinic has grown to more than 450 employees in 10 main ophthalmology-based offices, nine optometric/optical offices and 25 outreach clinical sites. Doctors also perform surgery at 33 Iowa hospitals statewide.

Another major milestone for Swartz was developing a partnership with Dallas County Hospital in 2007, which led to the opening of three operating rooms in an outpatient surgery center. Three years later, the surgery center was acquired by the Wolfe Eye Clinic board and renamed Wolfe Surgery Center. Due to ongoing success and growth, Wolfe Surgery Center expanded to six operating rooms in a new building in 2019.

"No one outworked Kevin, I mean no one," said Randy Eckard, former chief operating officer who worked with Swartz for more than 20 years. "And it has been my honor and privilege to have worked with Kevin over the years. Simply a stellar leader in every sense."

Dr. Matthew Rauen added: "You will not meet a more genuine and down to earth individual."

While Swartz did oversee massive geographic expansion as CEO, he's most proud of

the people he works with. Wolfe Eye Clinic has 28 ophthalmologists and 18 optometrists on staff, and Swartz played a key role in recruiting a great many of them. With rare exception, the doctors who join the clinic stay throughout their careers.

For Swartz, people are the lifeblood of a business. It's the people who continue to push Wolfe Eye Clinic forward. And it's the people who will improve the business for the next 100 years.

"The doctors and staff we have are what I'm most proud of," Swartz said. "The quality of what we've been able to achieve has been great and the people we have now will be able to maintain the quality and grow what we have. The territory is great, and the market share is great, and if you bring good people together and you keep them working together, it's going to lead to even greater things."

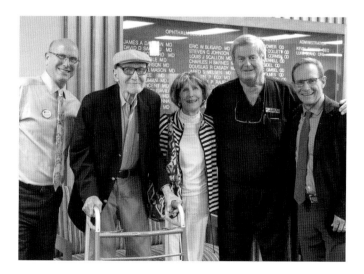

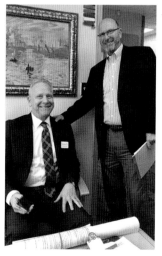

Left photo, left to right: Kevin Swartz, Dr. Russ Watt and his wife Marie Watt, Dr. James Davison and Dr. David Sagau at an open house event in 2019 celebrating 100 years of Wolfe Eye Clinic in Marshalltown.

Right photo, left: Randy Eckard, former chief operating officer, played a key partnership role in growth over the years with Swartz.

EDUCATION IN EYE CARE

Wolfe Eye Clinic has participated in training health care workers for years, likely starting with visiting eye surgeons learning cataract surgery techniques from founder Otis R. Wolfe. These informal types of knowledge sharing and surgical techniques continued for years as innovations emerged at the clinic. In the 1980s, more formal training activities began to occur. Wolfe Eye Clinic hosted optometry students for their quarterly rotations during the final year of training. The clinic also offered an optometry fellowship.

When the Iowa Legislature expanded the diagnostic optometry scope of practice in 1981, Wolfe Eye Clinic surgeons hosted laboratory training sessions on advanced examination techniques of the retina. In 1991, when the optometric scope of practice increased with respect to pharmacologic treatments, Wolfe Eye Clinic, with the assistance of the Pennsylvania College of Optometry, hosted courses for virtually all of Iowa's licensed optometrists, helping them gain their certification to prescribe pharmaceuticals.

Wolfe Eye Clinic participates with the University of Iowa College of Medicine and Des Moines Osteopathic College to provide clinical rotations to medical students. The students use this opportunity to gather ophthalmological experience that will help them in other specialties and determine whether they want to choose ophthalmology as a career path.

SPREADING RETINAL CARE INNOVATION

In 2016, Dr. Jared Nielsen, a retina specialist at Wolfe Eye Clinic, was approached by an academic medical center looking for help with its retina fellowship program. Wolfe Eye Clinic had respected retina surgeons, and it had the large patient base to support and train high-quality retina specialists. Nielsen was certainly interested, but regulatory hurdles halted the initial plan.

But the seed was already planted. Wolfe Eye Clinic's Board of Directors endorsed Dr. Nielsen's plan to launch its own two-year Vitreoretinal Fellowship Program in 2017, and it has quickly gained nationwide recognition. Fellows are involved in many surgeries and see a wide variety of patients. Heavy involvement in scientific clinical trials is also a huge plus. The University of Iowa is the only other organization in the state that offers such an opportunity, making Wolfe Eye Clinic the only privately owned institution to provide such vast learning for a fellow in Iowa.

Not only do fellows gain invaluable experience, practicing physicians learn a thing or two as well.

"It's great to be a mentor," Nielsen said. "It's been great to help people. When you are responsible for mentoring somebody, and you have them by your side all the time in the clinic and in the [operating room], it elevates the level of your practice. It pushes you to continue to provide the best care for patients and to help where we can."

Dr. James Davison, a cataract and refractive surgeon, added: "Seeing these young eager physicians learning and training with our surgeons has been

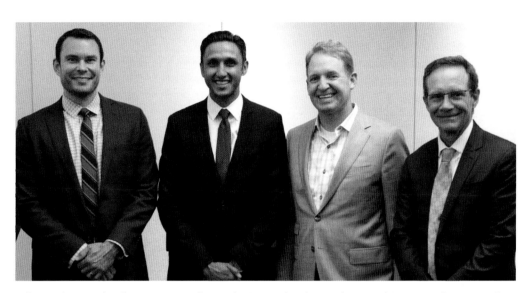

Left to Right: Dr. Kyle Alliman, Dr. Deepak Mangla, Dr. Jared Nielsen and Dr. David Saggau at the inaugural Wolfe Eye Clinic Retina Graduation Ceremony for Mangla.

inspirational for the rest of the clinic's surgeons and staff. The enthusiasm of the fellows and our surgeons has had a tremendous elevating effect on our entire organization."

Dr. Deepak Mangla, who was the first fellow in 2017, completed the fellowship in 2019. He's now a practicing retina specialist in Michigan. His experience was exceptionally positive. He said the opportunity was unlike any other in the United States.

"It was exactly what I was looking for," Mangla said. "I got to assist with more surgeries than any other fellow. I got to assist treating more patients than any other fellow. It was completely immersive. I had four mentors, who were really helpful in solving problems. You could see it from four different angles, and it was really beneficial to someone who was learning."

Mangla initially became intrigued by retina specialty because of the many advancements being made in the field. He wanted to be a part of something new. A native of Detroit, Mangla found his way to Wolfe Eye Clinic after his mentor during residency at Northwestern University connected him with Nielsen.

Speaking with his peers now, Mangla realizes Wolfe Eye Clinic provided him the perfect atmosphere to grow. "It was probably the best fellowship you could do," Mangla said. "The amount of exposure to surgery, the amount of supervised autonomy and the resources to pursue the things you wanted were amazing."

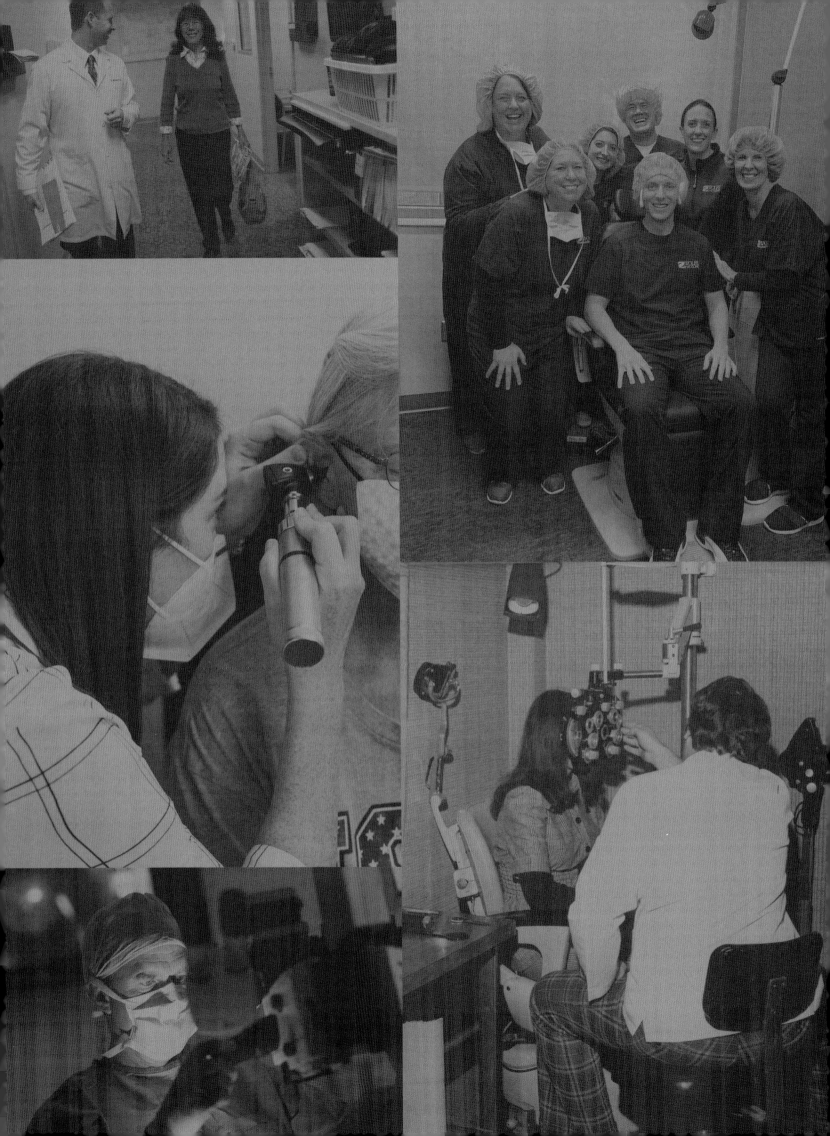

SUBSPECIALTIES

Just like other medical professions, ophthalmology has its own list of specific subspecialties. For many years in Wolfe Eye Clinic's history, physicians were tasked with treating all kinds of eye conditions. As technology and procedures advanced, the profession became more segmented as more expertise was required. Physicians were then hired to fill very specific needs.

Wolfe Eye Clinic provides quality care in a variety of subspecialties, from cataract to retina to LASIK. It's important to treat patients right, and the expert physicians at the clinic are on the leading edge of their respective fields.

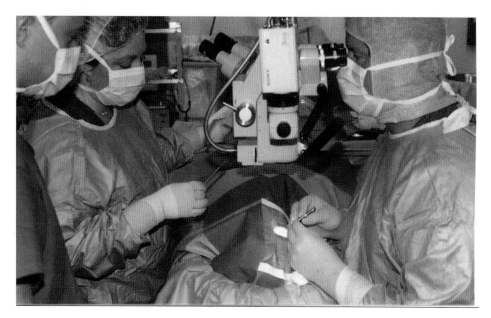

Cataract surgeries have come a long way since 1919, when Wolfe Eye Clinic was founded. Today, there are much-improved tools and procedures, some of which Wolfe Eye Clinic was first to adopt.

CATARACTS

Cataract surgery was the foundation on which Wolfe Eye Clinic was built. It remains important and is intricately woven throughout its history. From the very beginning, Dr. Otis R. Wolfe, who founded the business in 1919, sought to revolutionize cataract care to make the clinic a leader throughout the United States.

A cataract means the clouding of the natural lens of the eye. The natural lens is about the size of an M&M candy and sits just behind the colored iris. The lens is clear when a person is born. But with time, protein within the lens clumps together and starts to cloud. This clouding interferes with light passing through the eye, reducing the sharpness of the image reaching the retina. Over time, the cataract may grow larger and

cloud more of the lens, making it harder to see.

In the 1920s, procedures to correct cataracts actually removed the lens, but the process was messy. A surgeon typically made a small incision in the eye, cut the capsule open and stirred the soft nucleus inside, then sucked it out. But extracting the fluid sometimes caused more damage. This method worked pretty well on children with soft cataracts, but harder cataracts in adults could many times not be extracted safely this way.

In 1925, Wolfe performed the first cataract surgery using the Barraquer method, which was named after the famed Spanish ophthalmologist Dr. Ignacio Barraquer. The method used a suction apparatus that held on to the cataract, which

made it a much cleaner and less invasive procedure. A large incision was made about halfway around the eye where the white sclera meets the clear cornea and colored iris. The method used a vacuum device that he had invented, which was applied to the front surface of the cataractous lens. He then applied suction to that front surface while simultaneously pushing on the white sclera of the lower part of the eye. This method combined positive pressure from below and negative suction pressure

from above to lift the entire cataractous lens through the incision and out of the eye while an assistant lifted the cornea up so the lens could be delivered.

"It was innovative at the time," said CEO Kevin Swartz. "It was nothing like cataract surgery is now, but it was better than what was being done before."

That procedure became a defining mark for Wolfe Eye Clinic. By the 1930s, Wolfe had named the clinic Wolfe Cataract Clinic and saw patients across the United States. In 1930, Wolfe first performed intracapsular cataract surgery, a less invasive procedure, while he continued to use the aspiration technique on soft cataracts..

While cataract surgery was advancing, it still resulted in patients requiring thick glasses in order to see. And many times, a patient would have to be completely blind in order to undergo proper surgery. For the most part, cataract surgeries at Wolfe numbered in the hundreds every year,

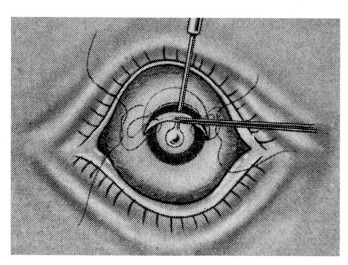

Figure 7 from Otis R. Wolfe's scientific paper showing a cataract being lifted by an erisphake cannula acting as a pneumatic suction forceps. (Otis R. Wolfe. 20 Years' experience with the Barraquer technic of cataract extraction. Journal International College Surgeons 1947; Vol. X No. 4: 398-403.)

rather than the thousands we see today. That's because the procedure only marginally improved vision.

All that changed in 1967, when phacoemulsification was invented — one of the first small-incision surgeries invented. Dr. Russell Watt and Dr. John Graether were among the first adopters of this successful technique in 1972. No longer were large incisions needed to remove the whole lens or the lens nucleus. Then, around 1976, there was an intermediate method available where a large incision was made and the nucleus of the cataract expressed by exerting external pressure on the globe. The large incision left the eye vulnerable to complications during surgery and required many stitches to close and more time to stabilize and heal. But the early adopters at Wolfe stuck with the newest technique.

Phacoemulsification was a new technique that utilized a new instrument that transmitted ultrasonic energy and

simultaneous vacuum to the cataractous lens substance through a very small needle. The lens substance was evacuated from the clear lining of the lens, which remained in the eye. The surgeon then removed the fluid. An incision was still required to introduce surgical tools, but it was much less invasive.

In 1975, Wolfe Eye Clinic performed its first lens implant surgery, which replaced the cloudy lens with an artificial lens. This helped patients restore vision more consistently after surgery, a huge advancement still used today, albeit with better quality artificial lens. It was considered particularly risky for the time, and Graether estimated that only about 10% of ophthalmologists were doing it. But Wolfe Eye Clinic had low complication rates thanks to its dedicated surgeons.

When Gov. Robert Ray, the popular Iowa politician, approached Graether in 1981 wanting the surgery, it caused some controversy in the ophthalmology field.

"Other clinics told him, 'No, don't have an implant. It's too dangerous,'" Greather said. "But we had a good reputation, and a low complication rate."

The surgery was an overwhelming success, and it helped springboard Wolfe Eye Clinic as a business.

Cataract surgeries continued to advance over the next decade. Graether co-invented the continuous tear capsulotomy in 1985, which is still the standard technique used throughout the world. That same year, Graether said Wolfe Eye Clinic performed more cataract surgeries than the entire state of Rhode Island — a testament to how well patients regarded Wolfe Eye Clinic.

"Here, we were considered rural, and here was Providence, Rhode Island, which is obviously not rural," Graether said. "We were doing more surgeries in Marshalltown, Iowa, than they were doing in Providence, Rhode Island. It was rather interesting."

The advancements in cataract surgeries in the 1980s were integral in Wolfe Eye Clinic's growth as a business. Demand for these procedures exploded, and locations were opened in West Des Moines, Fort Dodge, Cedar Falls, Cedar Rapids and more.

"The modern cataract procedure is really what allowed us to grow," Swartz

said, "That procedure became better and better, and more people were able to do it, and we seized on the opportunity."

In 1988, Wolfe Eye Clinic used the first foldable intraocular implanted lens for cataracts. In 1991 the federal government allowed co-management of postoperative care with ophthalmologists and optometrists so that patients would not have to travel back to their surgeons for checkups after surgery. Eyedrop topical anesthesia was introduced for cataract surgery in 1992. By 1999, cataract surgeries were extremely common. Thousands of patients were being treated every year. By 2000, Wolfe Eye Clinic had performed 100,000 cataract procedures.

The 21st century saw more marginal advancements in cataract care. Multifocal IOLs were introduced in 2003 and Toric IOLs were first used at Wolfe Eye Clinic in 2006, which corrected astigmatism during cataract surgery.

To date, Wolfe Eye Clinic has performed more 200,000 cataract surgeries over the course of its history, restoring sight and providing a new lease on life for many. Improvements in cataract surgery developed at Wolfe Eye Clinic often became the standard of care nationwide and globally.

A cataract is a clouding of the eye lens, resulting in blurred vision. Dr. Peter Rhee is shown here examining a patient's eye.

HEALTH

Cornea transplants restore vision

Not considered 'common' yet but many Iowans have had one

By Jan Mathew
Gazette Lifestyle writer

For most of her 42 years, vision for Barb Colehour was like looking "through a glass that was covered with fog." Keratoconus, an eye disease in which the center of the cornea becomes thin and cone-shaped, began destroying her vision at age 9.

Then in 1983, Colehour, of Mount Vernon, became one of 160 Iowans to undergo a cornea transplant.

"My vision is so much better than it ever was before," she reports. "The little bit of blurriness I do have I don't even notice."

If it were not for the Iowa Lions Eye Bank in Iowa City and the widespread practice of cornea transplants, conditions such as Colehour's would eventually have deteriorated to blindness. Since the eye bank was established in 1955, about 2,150 persons have received cornea transplants at University of Iowa Hospitals and Clinics.

Corneas are donated after a person dies. Donations from the Cedar Rapids area have increased greatly in the past several years, due largely to the efforts of St. Luke's and Mercy Hospital nurses, according to Don Pfeiler, who serves as statewide coordinator for the eye bank. In the 1970s, when Pfeiler was waiting for two corneas, only about 16 to 20 eyes were donated from Cedar Rapids. In 1984, this number was up to 120 donations.

"The key to (increasing donations) is having the nurse convinced that she should ask the family if they've considered a donation," says Pfeiler, 2348 Linden Drive SE.

"We think that families that do donate are able to lower their stress level at the time of a loved one's death, because their mind begins to switch from the negative to the positive. Something's living on, and they're doing some good."

COMPARED TO other procedures, such as cataract surgery, cornea transplants are rare, according to Dr. John Graether, an eye surgeon at Wolfe Clinic, Marshalltown. The clinic performs 26 cornea graphs (transplants) annually, compared to 3,000 cataract surgeries.

"That's because the indications for cornea transplants are relatively rare, and cataracts are a common disease," Graether explains.

The cornea is the clear, transparent dome-shaped structure at the front of the eye. In addition to keratoconus, Fuchs' dystrophy — a condition where the cornea loses cells critical to clarity and becomes cloudy and thickened — is another common reason for cornea transplants. Transplants also can correct scarring from cataract surgery and accidental injuries.

"Transplants work in cases where the retina still functions well," says Dr. Jay Krachmer, a U of I Hospitals ophthalmologist and medical director of the eye bank. "By giving the person a

Corneal transplantation

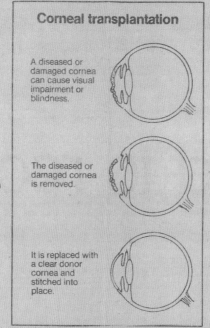

A diseased or damaged cornea can cause visual impairment or blindness.

The diseased or damaged cornea is removed.

It is replaced with a clear donor cornea and stitched into place.

clearer window, better vision could be the result. We're able to obtain a clear cornea in 95 percent of the cases."

Krachmer describes the surgical procedure as "fairly straightforward." A sharp, cylindrical instrument similiar to a cookie cutter is used to remove both the donor cornea and the patient's cornea. The donated cornea is then sewn into place with sutures finer than human hair. The patient is awake during the 90-minute surgery and usually is hospitalized for only 48 hours. Insurance covers the average cost, which is $2,500.

By comparison, the recovery period is quite extensive, according to surgeons. Healing takes a long time because the cornea contains no blood vessels, and sutures remain in the eye for up to a year, according to Graether. "The patient will see better immediately (following surgery), but maximum vision doesn't return until the sutures are removed."

Before his two cornea transplants, Pfeiler had great difficulty driving, reading or being outdoors in the sunlight. His condition, keratoconus, had deteriorated to the point where he could not wear contacts. "The contacts used to pop out of my eye when it was windy," he recalls. "The edges of the contacts couldn't lie on the cornea because it was too curved."

Following his two transplants in 1975 and 1976, Pfeiler's eyesight eventually returned to normal. "I knew a cornea transplant was necessary to save my sight. With contacts, my vision is now 20-20, and there's nothing that I can't do."

There is only a 10 percent chance that the body will reject the cornea, says Graether. Signs of rejection — decreased vision, redness and discomfort — generally can be reversed with medication.

Prior to surgery, most patients spend at least some time on a cornea tissue waiting list. Waiting often is the most difficult part of the entire procedure.

"Waiting caused the greatest anxiety," says Pfeiler. "There's always the uncertainty of *when* it will happen."

Pfeiler spent one year on a waiting list for his first cornea transplant, and several months for the second one. Doctors generally tell patients to expect to wait six or seven months.

The Lions Eye Bank hopes to cut the number on the waiting list from 100 to 25 persons, and limit the waiting period to 90 days.

AN UNUSUAL circumstance ended the limbo for one of Graether's patients, Doug Stover of Marshalltown. Previously treated with contacts, Stover's condition (keratoconus) had progressed rapidly and suddenly, the doctor says. Stover, 31, was on a cornea waiting list when his father died of a heart attack last October. On Oct. 11, Graether replaced Stover's diseased cornea with his father's. It was Graether's first surgery involving father and son.

"The probability (of a relative's cornea being transplanted) is so astronomically small because of the timing," says Graether. "It's also unusual to have a relative who would die at a young enough age with a suitable cornea."

"I could've waited for another cornea but I thought of how it would've pleased Dad," Stover said in a recent interview. "We just knew Dad would be happy about it. He was just that type of person."

Tissue often is taken from donors who died in late middle age, and some transplanted corneas that are now more than 100 years old are still helping patients see, according to Krachmer.

Cornea removal is optimal within four or five hours after death, and surgery should be performed within 48 hours, Graether adds. Recent advances have made it possible to store tissue for several days.

Persons who are interested in donating their corneas may request a donor card from the Iowa Lions Eye Bank, University of Iowa Hospitals and Clinics. According to the eye bank, it is crucial to notify relatives of a decision to donate tissue. If a donor card has not been filled out, relatives may sign a consent form at the time of death.

Wolfe Eye Clinic was one of the first in the state to perform cornea transplants in the 1960s, saving the vision of countless Iowans.

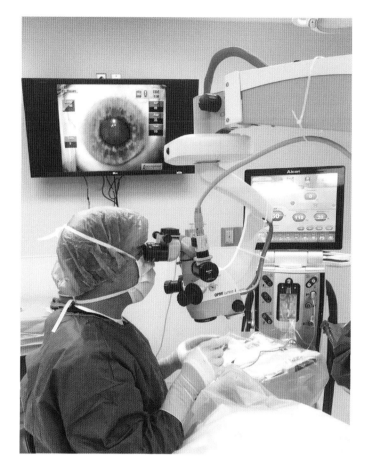

The cornea is your eye's clear, protective outer layer.

CORNEA DISEASE AND SURGERY

Corneas are an essential part of the eye structure. They are the eye's outermost layer — the clear, dome-shaped surface that covers the front of the eye. Any type of damage or obstruction blocks or bends how light enters the eye, ultimately blocking vision.

As early as the 1960s, Wolfe Eye Clinic was treating various ailments related to the cornea.

Corneal transplants were first performed at the clinic in 1960. Before the time of subspecializing, every physician helped in a range of surgeries. Cornea care was a big part of that.

"I did a lot of retinal surgery when I joined the clinic," said Dr. John Graether, who joined in 1962. "I had done a couple of cornea transplants and Dr. Russ

Watt had some experience there so we ultimately took on transplant surgery as well. Basically, we were offering pretty much a comprehensive range of surgical options for our patients."

The first full-time cornea specialist was Dr. Steve Johnson in the early 1990s. He joined when Wolfe Eye Clinic was undergoing significant change as subspecialties became more popular.

"We had [Johnson] come down [to Des Moines] and specialize in cornea," Dr. James Davison, who joined in 1980, said. "We were getting more specialized with different specialties. And things continued to change within all specialties like cornea, for example, so that full thickness corneal transplants are now rarely needed. They have been largely replaced

by other procedures such as DSAEK and DMEK, which replace only part of the cornea. They are faster and safer to perform and allow much faster recovery and better vision."

In the mid-1990s, Johnson was the first physician at Wolfe Eye Clinic to perform PRK and LASIK surgery, which reshapes the cornea to improve vision. In 1999, Wolfe Eye Clinic was the first in central and eastern Iowa to perform the intracorneal rings procedure, which affects the cornea's curvature, to correct nearsightedness.

Wolfe Eye Clinic can treat several corneal diseases today, including conjunctivitis (pink eye), keratoconus, dry eye, Fuchs' corneal dystrophy, corneal anterior basement dystrophy, corneal injuries and corneal abrasions, at most of its main offices.

GLAUCOMA

Glaucoma is a relatively common eye disease that gradually steals vision, sometimes without noticeable sight loss for many years. That's because it initially affects side or peripheral vision, which can be hard to notice. Glaucoma is a leading cause of blindness because it is so difficult to diagnose and control.

While today there are effective treatments to mitigate slowly advancing damage, that wasn't always the case. In the early 20th century, glaucoma would often lead to blindness as treatments were still coming of age.

Wolfe Eye Clinic has treated glaucoma for about 90 years. Its physicians — even its founder — have written articles on advanced glaucoma care, including surgical treatment during cataract procedures.

Dr. Otis R. Wolfe, the founder of the clinic, used to primarily treat cataract and glaucoma patients in his downtown Marshalltown office. From the outset, Wolfe worked closely with referring optometrists to provide the best patient care possible. Throughout the majority of the 20th century, optometrists weren't allowed

to treat patients for glaucoma or other diseases, even though they were crucial professionals in their local communities.

The ophthalmologists at Wolfe Eye Clinic have all been trained in the diagnosis, medical management and surgical treatment of glaucoma. But back before 1990, Iowa optometrists as well as optometrists from many other states had not been certified by their states to treat glaucoma or many other diseases with topical medications. The Wolfe ophthalmologists wanted to help Iowa optometrists

achieve their certification so that they could treat their patients more conveniently and closer to home. The Wolfe doctors were able to work with the Pennsylvania College of Optometry to design a curriculum and present seminars and training sessions that would allow certification upon completion and testing.

"Optometrists were able to achieve a legislative victory and treat patients for glaucoma and topical diseases," Dr. John Graether said. "Prior to that, they hadn't been able to do that at all; all they had achieved was just being able to dilate the eye. So again we stepped up."

Wolfe Eye Clinic was a leader in its own right as well. In 1985, Wolfe Eye Clinic doctors began using laser light to treat glaucoma. Lasers are still used today, albeit at a much more advanced level with computerized diagnostics. In 2003, Wolfe Eye Clinic performed its first Selective Laser Trabeculosplasty (SLT), a laser surgery used to treat glaucoma.

There are many ways to diagnose and treat glaucoma on an ongoing basis. Physicians at all Wolfe Eye Clinic locations are trained in proper care. Wolfe Eye Clinic also has glaucoma specialists, who are renowned experts in their field, on staff. Surgical treatments have evolved from trabeculectomies and laser to also include valves and several types of evolving minimally invasive glaucoma surgeries (MIGS).

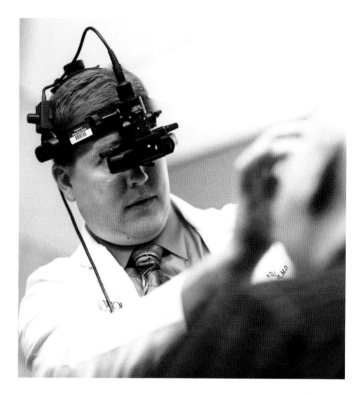

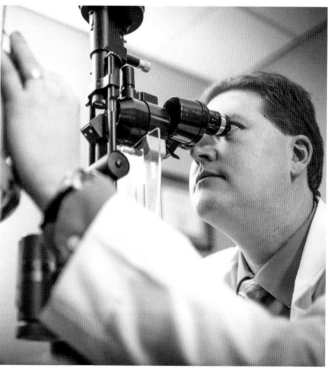

Glaucoma is the leading cause of blindness for those over 60. Wolfe Eye Clinic has been treating the disease almost as long as its been in existence. Dr. Ryan Vincent has been a glaucoma specialist with Wolfe Eye Clinic since 2014.

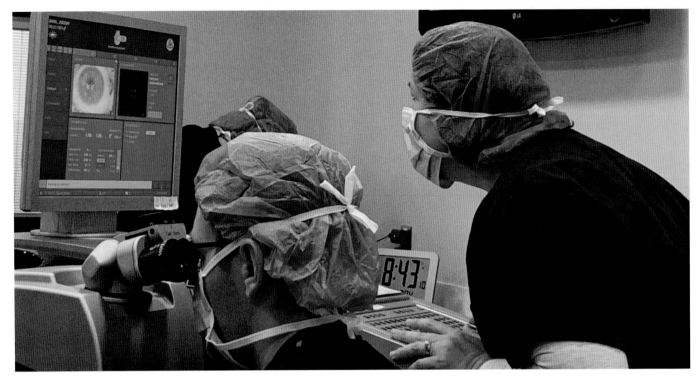

LASIK and refractive surgery change the shape of the dome-shaped clear tissue of the eye, helping patients be less reliant on glasses or contacts. Dr. Reid Turner and staff member Kim Padgett are shown here performing LASIK.

LASIK & REFRACTIVE SURGERY

Since it was discovered in the 1960s and came to prominence in the 1970s and '80s, refractive surgery, a broad term that includes Radial Keratometry, Photorefractive Keratectomy (PRK), LASIK and all-laser LASIK has changed millions of lives.

The procedure was performed with a metal blade in the early years. Surgeons precisely reshaped the cornea using radial cuts, vastly improving vision from common sight issues of nearsightedness, farsightedness and astigmatism.

Individuals who wore contacts or glasses now enjoyed a level of vision they never had before. Wolfe Eye Clinic performed its first refractive surgery, Radial Keratometry, in 1984.

In the 1990s, a new method was popularized that replaced a metal blade with an excimer laser — a precursor to the LASIK procedure we know today. Lasers were exceptionally precise, meaning eyesight could be improved beyond what was capable with a human hand.

In 1994, Wolfe Eye Clinic was the first in Iowa to acquire an excimer laser. Drs. Steve Johnson and Todd Gothard became investigators in FDA clinical trials for the device and its applications. In 1997, the clinic officially adopted the early LASIK procedure and switched to all-laser LASIK in 2002. Dr. James Davison was one of the initial Wolfe Eye Clinic physicians to perform LASIK. He said it was revolutionary for patients.

"It's transformative to patients," he said. "It's unbelievable.

What it does for people — it lets them have clear vision when they couldn't see before. They couldn't see their feet in the shower, they couldn't see their alarm clock, couldn't see television. If they lost their glasses, they couldn't see where they were going."

The tool was so well received, Wolfe Eye Clinic knew it was important to train as many people as possible to use it.

"We wanted to get this procedure out there into

several people's hands, so we trained each other and did more and more," Davison said. "The model of getting the best technology available and make it available to the patients who need it and want it and qualify for it, exposes them to a transformative experience."

There are two steps to a modern LASIK procedure. The first is the creation of the corneal flap. A laser creates a precise, thin flap of tissue that allows LASIK doctors to perform a more accurate procedure. For the second step, a surgeon utilizes the excimer laser, which gently breaks molecular bonds between cells, and reshapes the cornea. In all, the actual laser treatment takes less than 30 seconds per eye. Most patients experience a dramatic improvement in vision within hours or even minutes.

LASIK has now become a fairly routine procedure. The excimer laser used in LASIK has advanced with wave front and topography guided technology. These systems measure and capture the

unique visual distortions — similar to a "fingerprint" of your visual system. The detailed information is then converted to a map and is very precisely matched to your eye. The map can then be used to guide the laser to create a customized treatment for each individual.

Wolfe Eye Clinic has been one of the leaders in adapting those tools. The clinic has performed more than 32,000 refractive surgeries in its history, and the LASIK all-laser procedure is available in main clinics throughout Iowa, including surgery centers in West Des Moines and Cedar Rapids. Corneal Collagen Crosslinking surgery is also available at the centers. It stabilizes corneas that are weakening over time. That physical stabilization also stabilizes the refraction patients need to see clearly.

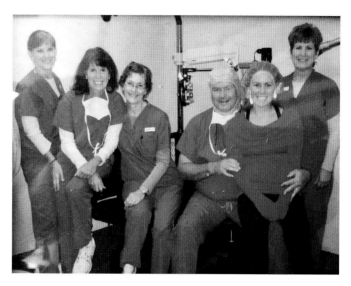

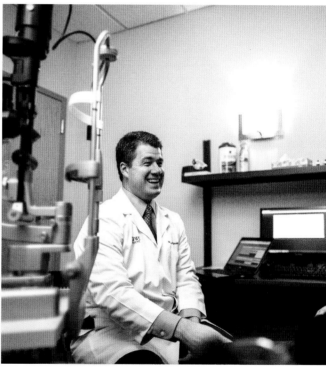

Top: Dr. James Davison featured here with his LASIK surgery team on the day of his daughter Megan's surgery.

Bottom: Dr. Matthew Rauen is one of many LASIK specialists at Wolfe Eye Clinic.

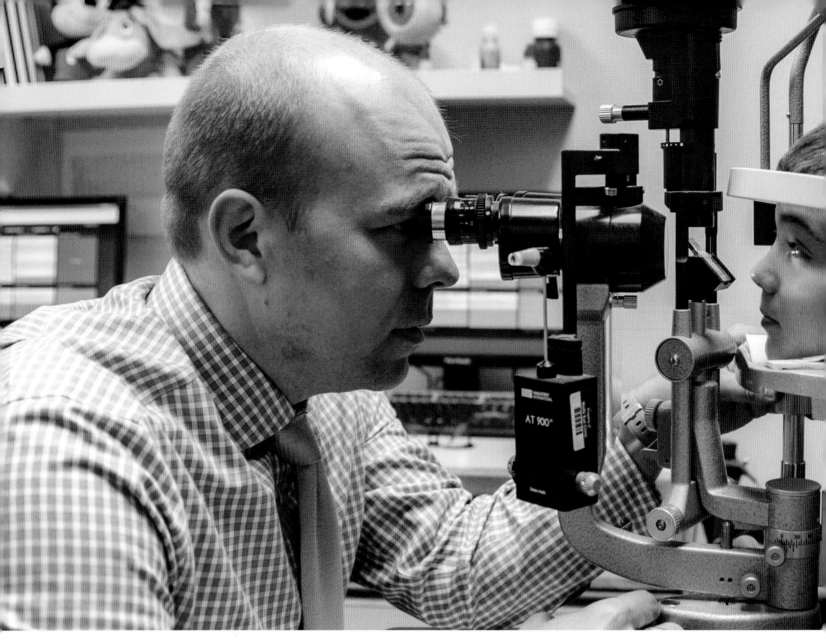

Dr. Derek Bitner, pediatric ophthalmologist, performs an exam on a patient.

PEDIATRIC OPHTHALMOLOGY

Pediatric ophthalmology, eye care for children, wasn't a subspecialty of its own at Wolfe Eye Clinic until 2000. Before, many ophthalmologists worked comprehensively, treating both adults and children in their day-to-day schedules.

That's what enticed Dr. Donny Suh to joined the clinic at the turn of the century. He saw there was an opportunity to build a subspecialty from the ground up. And fresh off his fellowship at the Johns Hopkins University College of Medicine, it was a challenge he was ready for.

"The Wolfe Eye Clinic was providing excellent service, but they had never had a pediatric ophthalmologist, and I was excited to take on the challenge of creating a whole new service

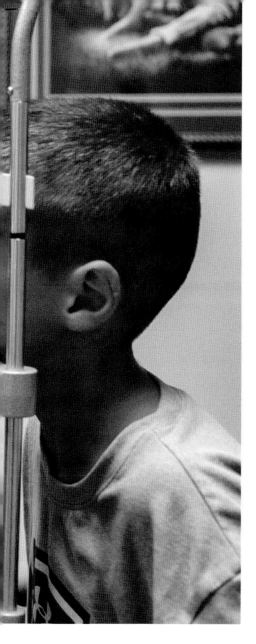

line," said Suh, who is now a pediatric ophthalmologist and adult strabismologist at the Children's Hospital and Medical Center in Omaha, Nebraska. "The clinic was basically a leader in ophthalmology, so I wanted to come in and make it the best pediatric clinic in the country."

Suh was located in the West Des Moines branch, which was just about to move into its first separate clinic space in 2004. Building the infrastructure took time. The pediatric service needed its own staff, its own equipment and its own room to grow. Thanks to the sterling Wolfe Eye Clinic reputation, the division took off in quick order, and Suh was the only physician overseeing the department for many years.

Wolfe Eye Clinic has been a longtime leader in pediatric research, joining the Pediatric Eye Disease Investigator Group in 2000. The organization administers studies for medical advancements in pediatric ophthalmology. The affiliation with PEDIG was an important one for Wolfe Eye Clinic, as it helped establish the pediatric ophthalmology department as a legitimate division.

"That was huge," Suh said. "That helped put us on the map. It helped us to be recognized and respected all across the country."

After 14 years at Wolfe Eye Clinic, Suh left in 2014, leaving a two-year gap until Dr. Derek Bitner joined the West Des Moines office in 2016. In the years since, the pediatric ophthalmology department has significantly grown in size thanks to a merger with Des Moines' Children's Eye Clinic in 2019, adding an experienced pediatric ophthalmologist in Dr. Jean Spencer to the staff. Cedar Rapids also has a pediatric ophthalmology subspecialty, added by Dr. Anne Langguth.

The association with PEDIG continues to be a strong partnership for Wolfe Eye Clinic, which is considered a top-five recruiter for the organization's medical trials and has won numerous awards. PEDIG has administered dozens of studies.

Wolfe Eye Clinic has been a participant in more than half of them.

Wolfe Eye Clinic is dedicated to advancing its clinical care at every opportunity, which is why medical trials present such a fruitful opportunity. Wolfe Eye Care is also one of the few private practices to offer pediatric ophthalmology services, which means it has an obligation to provide the best care possible.

"In Central Iowa, there's nobody else that does this," Bitner said. "We try to see as many kids as we can to help them out. There's not a lot of private practices in this space, and I think that makes us really unique."

RETINA DISEASE AND SURGERY

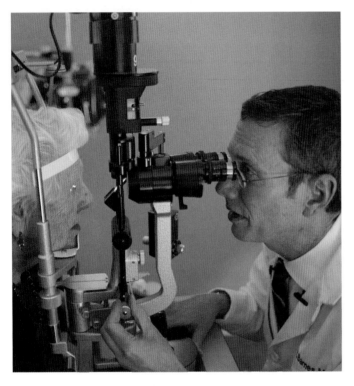

The retina is a sensory layer at the back of the eyeball that connects to the optic nerve, allowing you to see light and shapes. Dr. Charles Barnes in Cedar Rapids is one of many retina specialists at Wolfe Eye Clinic.

The retina is an unassuming thin layer of tissue located on the back wall of the eye. While it doesn't look like much, the retina plays a vital role in vision. It is composed of millions of light-sensitive cells connected with nerve fibers that allow light entering the eye to be converted into electrical impulses. These impulses are sent to the brain via the optic nerve. The retina is the connector between these nerve impulses and the brain via the optic nerve, allowing us to see.

Because of its complexity and importance, the retina requires special care for both common and complex problems, including macular degeneration, diabetic eye disease, retina detachment and macular holes. Wolfe Eye Clinic has been a nationwide leader in retina care and innovation for more than 60 years.

The advancement dates back to the 1960s, when Dr. Otis D. Wolfe, Dr. Russell Wolfe, Dr. Russell Watt, Dr. John Graether and Dr. Russell Widner pushed each other to be the best ophthalmologists possible. That led to a rise in innovation and was integral in the clinic's statewide growth. For example, in 1965, xenon arc photocoagulation was first performed at Wolfe Eye Clinic. The procedure used a xenon arc laser to treat previously untreatable retina diseases.

Physicians throughout the 1960s, '70s and '80s didn't typically specialize. That meant Wolfe Eye Clinic ophthalmologists performed procedures in all parts of the eye. Drs. Watt and Graether spent extra time doing cornea work and Drs. Widner and Davison spent theirs doing retina. In the 1990s, the industry became more segmented. More specialization was needed to perform more technologically advanced and complex surgeries.

"When I trained there were very few subspecializing," Graether said. "Now some of the specialties like retina have become in such high demand that these people in retina do nothing but retina because the demand is so high for their skill."

Dr. David Saggau became the first retina specialist at Wolfe Eye Clinic in 1990, following a retinal fellowship with Cleveland Retina Associates. At first, Saggau had a hand in all kinds of specialties, but as Wolfe Eye Clinic grew and hired more physicians, Saggau transitioned to full-time retinal care by 1995.

"By that time, we were really the only group big enough in Iowa to retain that kind of differentiation and specialization," said Saggau, who was splitting time between Marshalltown and Des Moines. "Otherwise it's just the University of Iowa."

More physicians were added to the retina specialty in the 1990s, and procedures continued to advance as well, particularly for treatment of age-related macular degeneration — the leading cause of severe, permanent vision loss in people over 60. In 1999, the first use of transpupillary thermotherapy was used to treat specific forms of AMD. A year later, photodynamic therapy was added as a treatment option. By 2001, Wolfe Eye Clinic used the feeder vessel treatment with high-speed ICG angiography. In 2005, Wolfe Eye Clinic first used an intravitreous injection for the treatment of wet-type AMD.

Dr. Jared Nielson joined Wolfe Eye Clinic as a retina specialist in 2007. Nielson remembers it as a unique time for the treatment

of retinal diseases. A few years before, the first eye injections to treat retinal diseases were made available, revolutionizing retinal care.

"And that really opened up the possibility of treating all sorts of blinding disorders and retinal diseases that people used to universally lose vision from," Nielson said.

Nielson spearheaded an effort to participate in national retina medical trials and advance these groundbreaking procedures. When he arrived at Wolfe Eye Clinic, Dr. Donny Suh was already involved in pediatric ophthalmology research groups. It made sense for the retina specialty to do the same.

The focus was always on providing patients with the latest and best treatments they couldn't get anywhere else. Trials included treatments for macular degenerations, wet and dry diabetic eye diseases and more. These advancements helped separate Wolfe Eye Clinic from other retina providers throughout the country.

Retina procedures today are completely different than

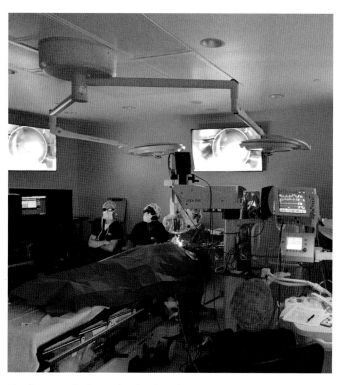

The first use of advanced technology for retina surgery in 2019 with use of the NGenuity equipment at Wolfe Surgery Center.

what they were 60 years ago. Advanced procedures such as pneumatic retinopexy (placing an air bubble in the eye to hold the retina in place) and intravitreal injections reduce the need for traditional surgery, making the restoration of vision for patients with retinal disease more successful than ever before. The small-incision, no-stitch vitrectomy surgery, first performed at Wolfe Eye Clinic in 2002, is minimally invasive and much more comfortable for the patient.

Wolfe Eye Clinic is a recognized national leader in retina treatments, providing complete retina services throughout the state. With seven retina specialists on hand, patients can have peace of mind knowing they are in the care of some of the best physicians in the country.

"We've been able to maintain a leadership position in the retina community here in Iowa," Nielson said. "We're always involved in what's new. It's exciting."

OCULOFACIAL PLASTICS

Oculoplastics, also known as oculofacial plastics, handles disease and surgery of the structures around the eye. This care has been a part of the Wolfe Eye Clinic story for several decades, beginning with most of the general ophthalmologists performing procedures to correct eyelid malfunctions of patients.

That expanded in 1978 with the arrival of Dr. Michael Hill, who specialized in otolaryngology, which refers to the surgery and management of conditions around the head and neck. Hill brought some of the first laser treatments for skin resurfacing and rejuvenation, while expanding the expertise of eyelid and brow surgical procedures offered at Wolfe Eye Clinic. At one time, it was reported that Dr. John Graether and Dr. Russell Watt performed eyeliner tattooing in the 1980s, which didn't seem to catch on. In 2005, Wolfe Eye Clinic recruited Dr. Doug Casady, a fellowship-trained oculofacial plastic surgeon, to join the clinic and build this subspecialty.

Today, oculofacial plastic surgeons at Wolfe Eye Clinic specialize in plastic and reconstructive surgery of the tissues around the eyes (forehead, eyebrows, eyelids, cheeks), lacrimal (tear) drainage system, and orbit (bones surrounding the eye). Because the position of the eyelid is vital to the health of the eye, many optometrists refer to our surgeons.

In 2019, Dr. Audrey Ko joined Casady as the clinic's second oculofacial plastic surgeon. Casady and Ko are two of only six oculofacial plastic surgeons with fellowship training in Iowa. Wolfe Eye Clinic offers oculofacial plastic and reconstructive surgery services at clinics located in Ames, Cedar Falls, Des Moines, Fort Dodge, Marshalltown and Ottumwa.

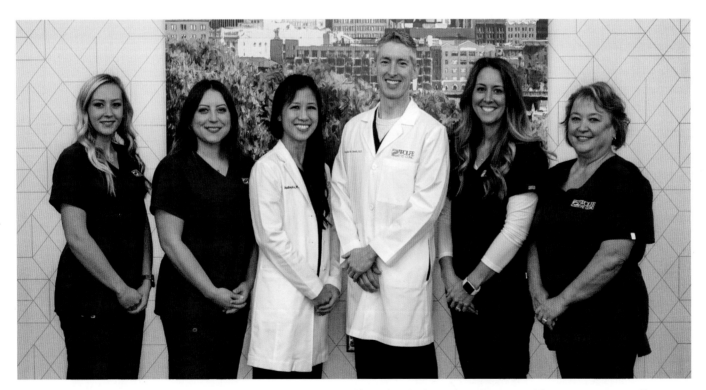

Dr. Audrey Ko and Dr. Douglas Casady, shown here with their team. While forms of oculoplastics have been around for many years at Wolfe Eye Clinic, today the clinic offers both medical and cosmetic procedures and has grown to two board-certified oculofacial plastic surgeons.

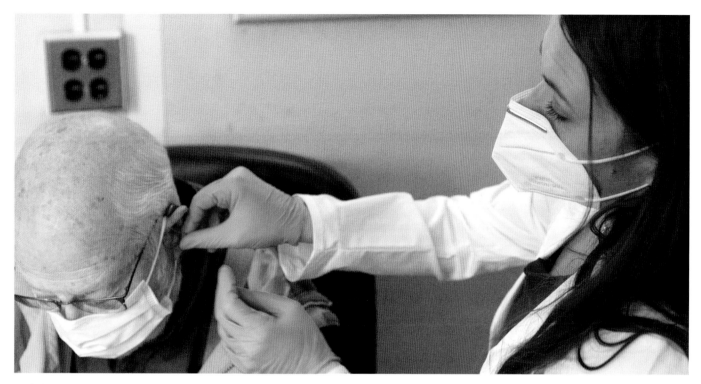

Audiologist Dr. Robyn Ritchey examines a patient's ears. Audiology has more than three decades of background at Wolfe Eye Clinic — even more considering ear, nose and throat care. Today, Wolfe Audiology serves people across the state.

AUDIOLOGY

Ear treatments were ingrained in Wolfe Eye Clinic from the beginning. When the clinic opened in 1919, care consisted of eyes, ears, nose and throat. Dr. Otis R. Wolfe, the founder, had previously trained under prominent eye, ear, nose and throat doctors in Chicago before moving to Marshalltown.

Wolfe Eye Clinic leaned toward eye care after it helped revolutionize cataract surgery in the 1920s and '30s and eventually phased out all ear, nose and throat services. They were reintroduced into the clinic in 1977, when an expansion of the Marshalltown office resulted in the addition of an ear, nose and throat specialty. Audiologists later joined the company, and they followed the same innovative mindset as their ophthalmologist co-workers.

In 1992, Bruce Vircks in the Wolfe Audiology department first used an implantable hearing device, called the Xomed implant. A year later, Vircks introduced Resound hearing aid technology, which is a more sophisticated hearing aid better attuned to the patient's specific need.

Wolfe Audiology is still an important part of the Wolfe Eye Clinic brand today. There are two licensed audiologists on staff, serving four Iowa cities: Ames, Cedar Falls, Des Moines and Marshalltown. Services include hearing testing, hearing aid fitting and tinnitus therapy. Like the Wolfe Eye Clinic itself, Wolfe Audiology is focused on patients first, working hard to develop relationships and top-quality care.

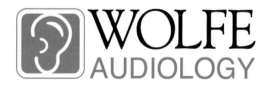

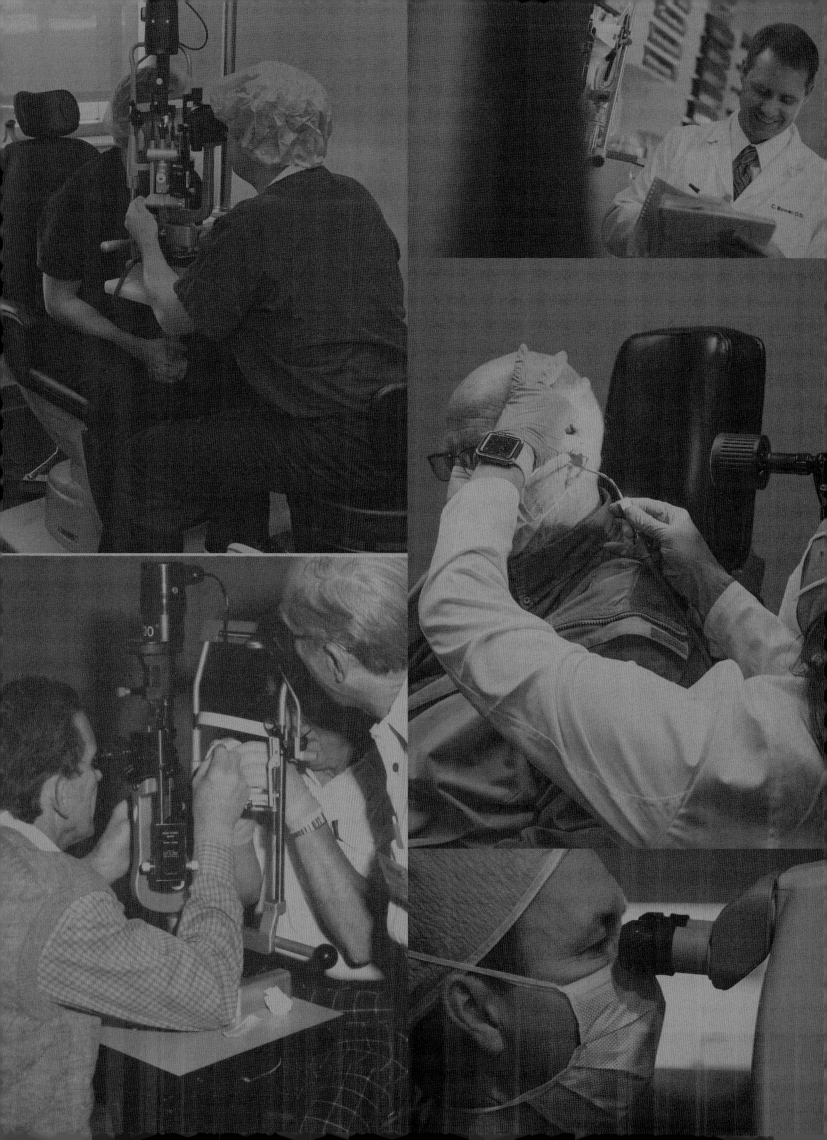

CLINICAL RESEARCH

and Medical Trials

CLINICAL TRIALS AND ADVANCING THE INDUSTRY

Becoming one of the nation's leaders in ophthalmic care and innovation doesn't happen by chance. Throughout the years, Wolfe Eye Clinic has taken steps to be on the cutting edge by taking part in top national research organizations and medical trials.

From the beginning, advancement was ingrained in Wolfe Eye Clinic's core mission.

Dr. Otis R. Wolfe, who founded the clinic in 1919, was one of the first in the United States to perform the Barraquer method of cataract surgery in the 1920s. He traveled to Spain to research the procedure under Dr. Ignacio Barraquer, the inventor of the method himself.

In the 1960s and '70s, Wolfe Eye Clinic was led by an innovative group of physicians. In 1972, the clinic was one of the first in the nation to receive a phacoemulsification machine to be used in an improved procedure to remove cataracts. Because of the controversial nature of the surgery, Wolfe Eye Clinic physicians trained with the phacoemulsifier many times before using it with real patients.

It was that aptness to try something new and advanced that helped Wolfe Eye Clinic boast one of the lowest complication rates of the phacoemulsification procedure, which was a particularly tricky surgery at the time and physicians around the country were wary to use it. Wolfe Eye Clinic saw it as an opportunity to advance the care they were providing.

"We actually bought the equipment when it was commercially available in 1972, and we decided that because of the controversial nature of the procedure, that we'd get used to it for a couple of months," said Dr. John Graether, one of the leading innovative surgeons in Wolfe Eye Clinic's history. "We quickly learned what operations were suitable for phacoemulsification and completed the first procedure in December that year, even though we had the equipment in September."

Graether has always been passionate about research and holds several patents of his own. He's written numerous papers and contributed to the advancement of the opthtalmology profession. His tool, the Graether Pupil Expander, was created in 1996 and is still used today.

Many of Wolfe Eye Clinic's research and trial methods of the 1960s and '70s were informal, but they helped set a precedent, eventually leading to a more formal approach with publications by Graether and his associates starting in the 1980s. Davison particularly enjoyed writing and publishing his observations and clinical series and was an investigator in the FDA clinical trials of the first apodized diffractive multifocal intraocular lens.

Opposite page: Wolfe Eye Clinic was one of the first in the state to perform phacoemulsification surgery in the 1970s, as this article in the Marshalltown Times-Republican describes.

Wolfe Clinic's 5,000th Phaco-Emulsification Brings Party

By LORRAINE SCHULTZ
(Staff Writer)

A surprise appreciation party, complete with a cake which read "Congratulations on Your 5,000th Phaco-Emulsification" was held earlier this week at the Marshalltown Area Community Hospital in honor of the Operating Room nurses and technicians who have assisted the Wolfe Clinic Eye Surgery Team.

Dr. Henry Wolfe, spokesman for the Wolfe Clinic, explains that the party was given "mostly to brag up the hospital and the job it's doing for us and for the community — and to make official note of the fact that the phaco-emulsification procedure for cataract removal, which we started doing in December of 1972, has been highly successful for us and has led to a great deal of growth for both the clinic and the hospital."

Dr. Russell Watt, senior surgeon on the four-member Wolfe eye surgery team, explains that the large number of phaco-emulsification cataract removal procedures has demanded an increase in the OR staff at the hospital, demanded an increase in records keeping and clerical personnel, and "put us in on the ground floor for even more sophisticated eye surgery procedures — in fact, is the background behind the fact that the Wolfe Clinic is now doing an ever-increasing number of lens implantations."

Revolutionary Procedure

Phaco-emulsification in 1972 was a revolutionary procedure for cataract removal: The patient could be up and about his or her business in three or four days rather than going through an agonizing six-week convalescence from cataract removal. Cataract removal accounted for about 300 surgeries a year at the Marshalltown hospital; that number was expected to increase to 500 in the first year. Currently the Wolfe team is performing on the average of eight eye surgeries a day (not all of which are phaco-emulsification, but it's the most frequently used procedure for cataract removal — others are still valid, and some patients will benefit from the conventional procedures).

Since 1972 the procedure has been modified somewhat, reports Dr. Watt, with ever-increasing sophistication of equipment and techniques which, of course, demand additional investment on the part of the hospital. "The hospital has been extremely cooperative in pro-

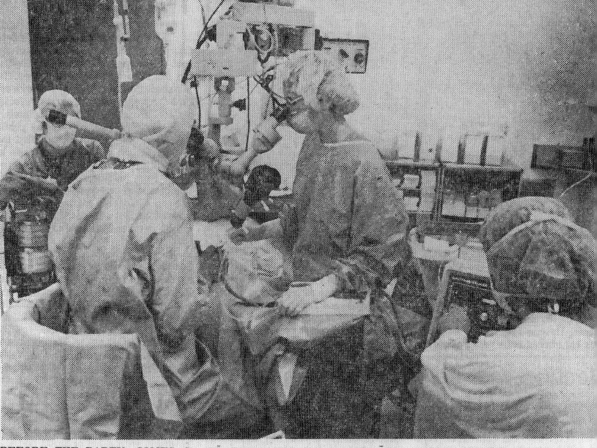

BEFORE THE PARTY...COMES the work...and the work, in this case, is completion of the 5,000th phaco-emulsification cataract removal by the Wolfe Clinic eye surgery team and the Marshalltown Area Community Hospital Operating Room team. Shown here, in the actual operating room situation, with a Des Moines woman, Blanche Taake, as the patient, are (from left to right) Mike Knight, anesthesiologist; Dr. Russell Watt, surgeon; Mrs. Jan Faber, RN, and Deb Mullen, monitoring the Kelman Phaco-Emulsification electronic console which is the "heart" of the surgical technique. Like all intra-ocular surgery, Dr. Watt is working through a powerful microscope, and in this case, utilizing a titanium-tipped handpiece which vibrates at 40,000 plus strokes per second, fragmenting the cataract, dissolving it (emulsifying and sucking it away with a pump-aspirator controlled by the console. After the surgery was over and the patient properly cared for, these four were able to join the party being thrown at the hospital by the Wolfe Clinic to show appreciation for the hospital staff's assistance in the performance of all eye surgeries. (Staff photo)

viding the Kelman equipment," says Dr. Watt. "Its support as demonstrated in its willingness to purchase additional equipment, at no small cost, is much appreciated by the Clinic."

Eight Trays Of Tools

Eight separate trays of hand-tools are required for a day's surgical schedule, with each tray worth between $3,500 and $7,000, says Dr. Watt. The original Kelman Cavitron console for photo-emulsification cost $40,000, but the hospital is on its third unit, each more sophisticated, more technically perfect, less apt to cause equipment problems, than the last — and each, of course, more expensive than the last, though old equipment can be sold when replaced and the investment can be amortized by the hospital.

When the local hospital and the Wolfe Clinic teamed up to do the first phaco-emulsification procedures here, Marshalltown was the only place in Iowa where the procedure was being done and one of only 34 sites in the nation. Drs. Otis Wolfe, John Graether, Russell Weidner, Gilbert Harris and Russell Watt were the only Iowans trained to perform the procedure; now the members of the Wolfe team are Drs. Watt, Graether, Weidner and Harris (with the loss of Dr. Gary Hedge earlier this year, the workload had increased proportionately, and in August a Dr. Davison from the Mayo Clinic, Rochester, Minn., fully qualified in phaco-emulsification, will be joining the team to ease the caseload).

OR Staff Feted

Members of the OR staff and anesthesia team who were all feted at the appreciation party included Janice Faber, who Dr. Watt credits with "a real feel for our equipment, what makes it tick, what we need, when we need it"; Catherine Swab, OR head nurse, who Dr. Watt says "keeps us in repair, keeps

Jolene Anderson, Michael Buller, J[...] Jensen, Sheryl Langenbau, Sha[...] Long, Mary Jo Parrott, Burgi Bartl[...] Nancy Swessinger, Darla Hanna, Le[...] Osten and Joyce Trickey.

Members of the anesthesia te[...] include Drs. William Wessels and Je[...] Winter, and Larry Bucher, Mich[...] Knight, Adra Maytag, Jan Rosenbl[...] and Cathy Wessels.

How do you tell when you've come[...] your 5000th phaco-emulsification? Dr. Watt reports that Mrs. Faber "lets [...] know whenever we turn 1,000 miles [...] each procedure — for instance we [...] just completed our 3,000th lens impl[...] tation, and although there are care[...] records kept here at the clinic, it's j[...] something that we doctors don't ta[...] note of unless the OR people comm[...] on it..."

SEMCO Board OKs Both Morning, Afternoon Kindergarten Sessions

LAUREL - The SEMCO Community School District Board of Education recently ratified the holding of both morning and afternoon kindergarten classes at Laurel in 1980-81, approved three teacher contracts and discussed possible closing of the junior high building by 1982-83.

In regard to the latter matter, it was decided that the third floor, due to recent building problems, could be closed off for the coming school year.

admit their holders to all home basketball, football and wrestling events. The price for conference games was set at $2 per event for adults and $1 per event for students.

Also, it was voted that participants in the Red Cross swimming lessons should be assessed $3 each at registration. The program this year will include pre-school children, and the total cost for the district is estimated at $900.

Purchase of a water purification

GROUNDBREAKING CLINICAL TRIALS

While researching and conducting FDA-sponsored clinical trials for devices and intraocular lenses has been a part of Wolfe Eye Clinic throughout the 20th century, a more formal partnership took shape in 2000. That year, Dr. Donny Suh joined as the clinic's first pediatric ophthalmologist, and he had a vision to create one of the strongest pediatric ophthalmology departments in the country.

To achieve the goal, Wolfe Eye Clinic partnered with the Pediatric Eye Disease Investigator Group (PEDIG), a national organization that administers clinical trials for child eye care and publishes results. In the two decades since, Wolfe Eye Clinic has won numerous national awards while gaining mentions in critical research papers. The clinic was also tabbed as a top-five medical trial site by PEDIG.

The benefits of participating in trials are twofold. One, physicians use instruments, procedures and drugs before they become commercially available, helping build familiarity. Two, patients receive some of the best care possible before it is available widely. These clinical trials are typically the final step of research prior to widespread release, meaning treatments have already been extensively tested and deemed safe.

"A lot of the studies we have done have altered the way we treat patients," said Dr. Derek Bitner, who joined Wolfe Eye Clinic in 2016 in the pediatric opthtalmology department. "So it keeps you on the leading edge."

Wolfe Eye Clinic strengthened its affiliation with medical trials when Dr. Jared Nielsen joined in 2007. A retina specialist, Nielsen was passionate about research and providing top care to patients. Because Suh was already working with PEDIG, it made sense for the retina department to get involved as well.

The first few studies focused on Lucentis, a treatment option for age-related macular degeneration (AMD), as well as treatments for diabetes and retinal vein occlusions.

"It started kind of slow," Nielsen said. "But it enabled us to get our feet wet and learn the ropes involved in retina clinical trials."

A year later, Wolfe Eye Clinic became involved with the Diabetic Retinopathy Clinical Research Network (DRCR.net), a collaborative network funded by the National Institute of Health that administers clinical trials for diabetic retinopathy, diabetic macular edema and related conditions. By 2009, clinical trials became such a big part of Wolfe Eye Clinic that it hired a full-time coordinator.

Quickly, Wolfe Eye Clinic became one of DRCR.net's best sites, helping run multiple trials for AMD and both wet and dry diabetic eye disease.

"From there, things began to move ahead," Nielsen said. "We're never involved in any trials unless they have something to offer the patient that they can't get anywhere else. Our trials are designed to look at having better outcomes, decreased treatment burden and trying to help patients see better. And it's been great. We're always involved in what's new." Since 2007 over 40 retina clinical trials have been conducted at Wolfe Eye Clinic, which has become acknowledged as a leading retina clinical trial center.

For example, a new drug was released in 2019 to treat wet AMD. Wolfe Eye Clinic had already been using the drug for four years at that point. Patients and doctors were familiar with its usage and effects.

Wolfe Eye Clinic has also been on the leading edge in using new tools for a number of different subspecialties. For LASIK, the clinic was the first in Iowa to obtain the Allegretto Wave Excimer Laser (2007), Wavelight FS200 laser (2011) and the Wavelight EX500 Excimer Laser (2015). Wolfe Eye Clinic was also the first in Iowa to use the LenSx laser in 2012 to

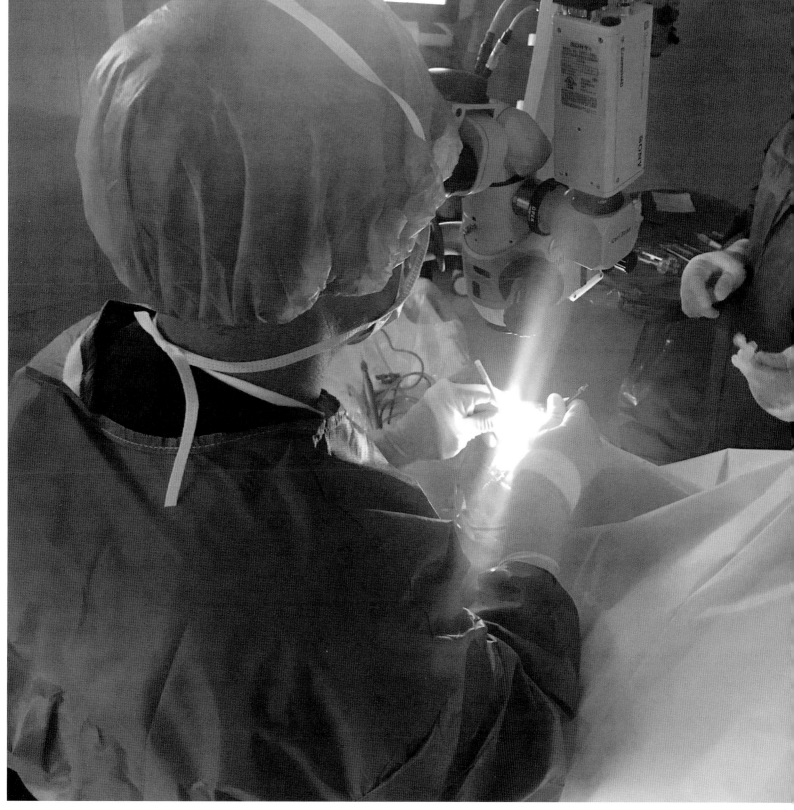

Wolfe Eye Clinic enrolls in all kinds of clinical trials, giving patients the latest in care while staying up to date on the best technology and procedures.

treat cataracts. The clinic was also the first site in Iowa to use the NGenuity 3D visualization for retina surgery in 2017.

"We enjoy staying on the leading edge of advancements in our specialty with the hope that they can make a difference for patients, from when we start investigating these advancements to when we start using them for patients," CEO Kevin Swartz said. "It's something we all get excited about."

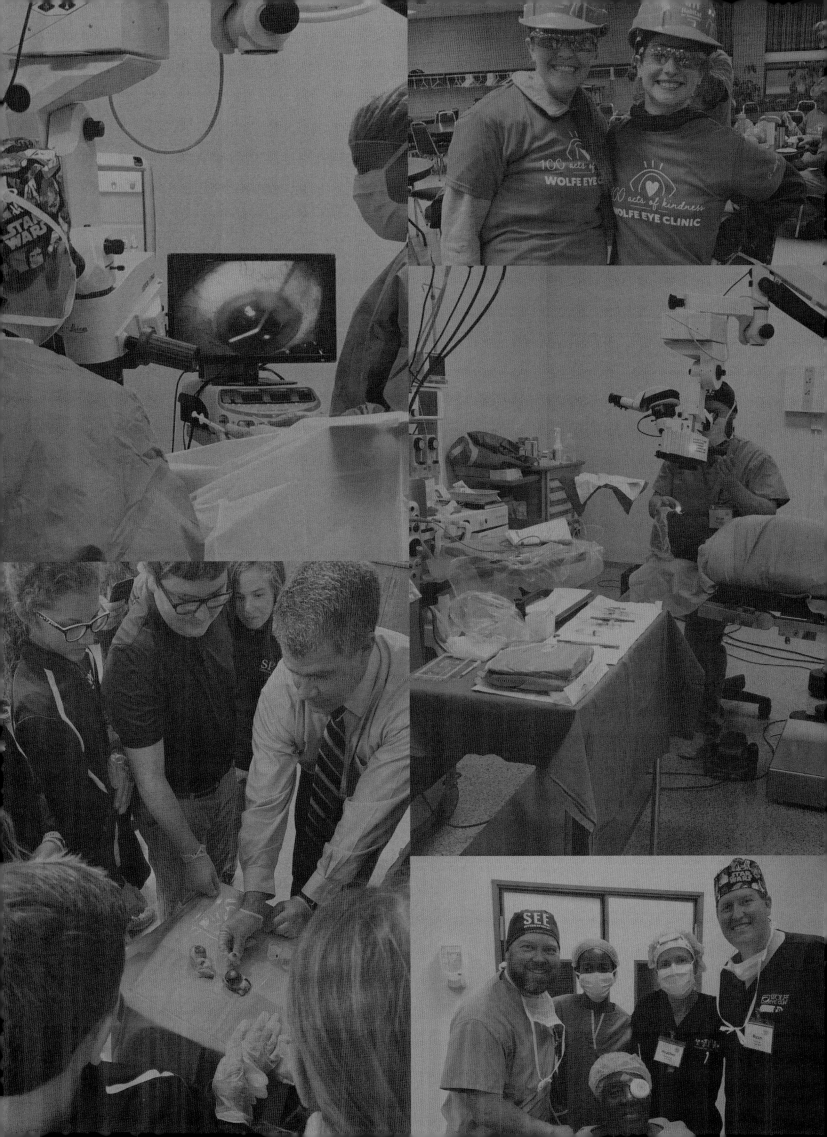

WOLFE
FOUNDATION

a Culture of Giving Back

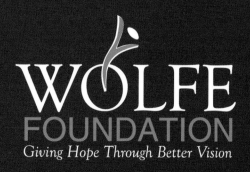

WOLFE
FOUNDATION
Giving Hope Through Better Vision

Yucatan Partners Members In City Vis

By MARY DOOLEY
(Staff Writer)

As part of the Iowa-Yucatan Partners of the Americas project, two Partners committee chairmen visited Marshalltown Thursday to discuss the progress and future direction of the various projects the Partners have undertaken in the past year.

The Partners program, originated by the U.S. Agency for International Development, provides for direct contact between people in the U.S. and Latin American countries and exchanges of technical and cultural resources. Iowa was paired with the Yucatan Peninsula, and has sent experts to assist in developing new wells, teaching natives how to clear land, raise new crops and care for their sick. Yucatan craftsmen, artists, dance troupes and students have come to Iowa to share their culture and heritage. During this school year, Mauricio Rodriguez of Merida, Yucatan, has served as a teacher-aide in Spanish language classes at Marshalltown High School, where he is also been a part-time student.

Eye Care Program

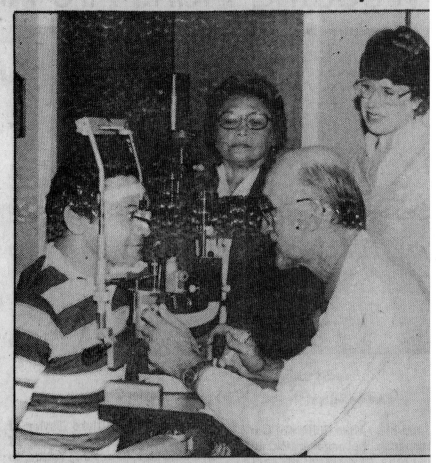

EXPERIENCING WOLFE CLINIC facilities first-hand, Dr. Salem of the Yucatan Peninsula, chairperson of the Iowa-Yu Peninsula Partners Public Health Committee, has his ey

Wolfe Eye Clinic physicians sometimes travel to other countries to provide care to at-risk groups.

A CULTURE OF PHILANTHROPY

Wolfe Eye Clinic has operated with compassion for those in need for more than 100 years. It's that mission that inspired visionary eye doctor Otis R. Wolfe, who founded the clinic in 1919, to create the Wolfe Cataract Foundation in 1936 — a time when Wolfe Eye Clinic was establishing itself as a national leader in ophthalmology.

The Wolfe Cataract Foundation included assistance and care for those who were facing loss of sight and simply could not afford the cost of treatment. Wolfe would often donate his time and resources for those who didn't have the funds or government assistance to pay for much-needed eye procedures.

The initial funding source for the Foundation was Wolfe's farmland in Kansas. He donated his acreages to the upstart nonprofit in order to provide the capital necessary to achieve his mission. In the first few decades of the new entity many of the Foundation patients were farm laborers. They didn't have the means to travel to the University of Iowa, where medical students in training often performed procedures at lower costs.

"Early on, the Foundation did a lot of that — taking care of indigent patients," CEO Kevin Swartz said. "The Foundation has continued to evolve and support a variety of patients and causes over time, so it's been a passion for us for many years."

Later renamed Wolfe Foundation, it went on to contribute to education

The original visions for the Foundation were simple but powerful:

- Provide charitable eye care to the needy.

- Support ophthalmic research and education.

by permanently funding an endowed lecture series for ophthalmologists across the Midwest hosted at the University of Iowa College of Medicine's Department of Ophthalmology and Visual Sciences.

Starting in 1969, the Wolfe Foundation Lecture has been delivered annually by some of the most distinguished ophthalmologists in the world. It has become one of the most prestigious ophthalmic lectureships and a cornerstone of the education program of the department. Two physicians from Wolfe Eye Clinic have given

lectures as a part of the series: Dr. John Graether (2004) and Dr. James Davison (2009), both revolutionary ophthalmologists.

In the 1970s and '80s, funds from the Wolfe Foundation helped Wolfe Eye Clinic conduct important research to advance the field of ophthalmology. But with a change in tax law that precluded funding of its own research, the Wolfe Foundation has instead donated money to outside ophthalmic research organizations to continue innovation in the field.

"It's been a really good organization for needy patients,"

Swartz said. "Some of the work it does has changed since the beginning, but it's been an important part of Wolfe's history for many years."

Giving back continues

The Wolfe Foundation has indeed evolved throughout the years, but it still operates with the same vision Wolfe put forth over 80 years ago. More than 95% of investments from compassionate donors go directly to the Foundation's mission — 75% for patient care, 20% to education and research.

Wolfe Eye Clinic physicians partner with the Foundation to donate their surgical time and other professional services, which leverages contributions to touch even more lives. The majority of Foundation dollars go directly to patient health expenditures.

The types of patients the Foundation helps have changed over the course of time as well. Medicaid was created in 1965, providing health insurance for most low-income patients.

But there is still a need among immigrant populations — a group of people who contribute greatly to the Iowa economy — and other underserved groups of people. Improved eyesight can change the course of someone's life, which ultimately can benefit local communities.

"The [Foundation] system does a good job of helping patients with vision problems, and that often helps them become employable and able to help themselves" Swartz said.

The cost of drugs and other treatment has increased in recent years, making the Foundation's mission even more important, particularly with older Americans. Age-related eye diseases are the leading cause of vision impairment and blindness in the United States. As the baby-boomer generation ages, more Americans than ever are being affected by age-related eye diseases such as macular degeneration, cataract, diabetic eye disease and glaucoma.

As our population ages, the number of people with age-related eye disease and the vision impairment that results is expected to double within the next two decades. And it is estimated that half of all age-related blindness could be prevented with access to timely evaluation and treatment. New technology and drug therapies have made treating these diseases much more successful. However, the cost associated with these treatments many times put them out of reach for uninsured or underinsured individuals.

The Wolfe Foundation, thanks to its dedicated and passionate donors, helps to fill that essential need.

"Wolfe Foundation helps people who don't have health insurance and don't fit into the Medicaid program and thus can't afford to have surgery," Swartz said. "Wolfe surgeons donate their time as surgeons and the Foundation helps pay other costs including hospital and anesthesia bills. Those are

amazing opportunities that we have at Wolfe Eye Clinic to additionally help people who otherwise could not achieve the medical cures that they need."

In addition to patient care and education, Wolfe Foundation supports eye-related organizations like Prevent Blindness Iowa and the American Diabetes Association. Funds are also provided for physicians to travel to underdeveloped nations. For example, Dr. Ryan Vincent traveled to Jamaica in 2019 to provide cataract and glaucoma surgery to those in need. Vincent helped reduce the local surgery waiting list by six months.

The Wolfe Foundation donated nearly $200,000 worth of services in 2019. Treatments helped restore vision that had been reduced by problems such as glaucoma, retina or corneal disease, in addition to helping patients in need with glasses and other eye-related expenses.

Opposite page: Dr. Ryan Vincent is pictured on a recent mission trip. Wolfe Eye Clinic has a long history of providing care to those in need, particularly through the Wolfe Foundation and the volunteerism of physicians.

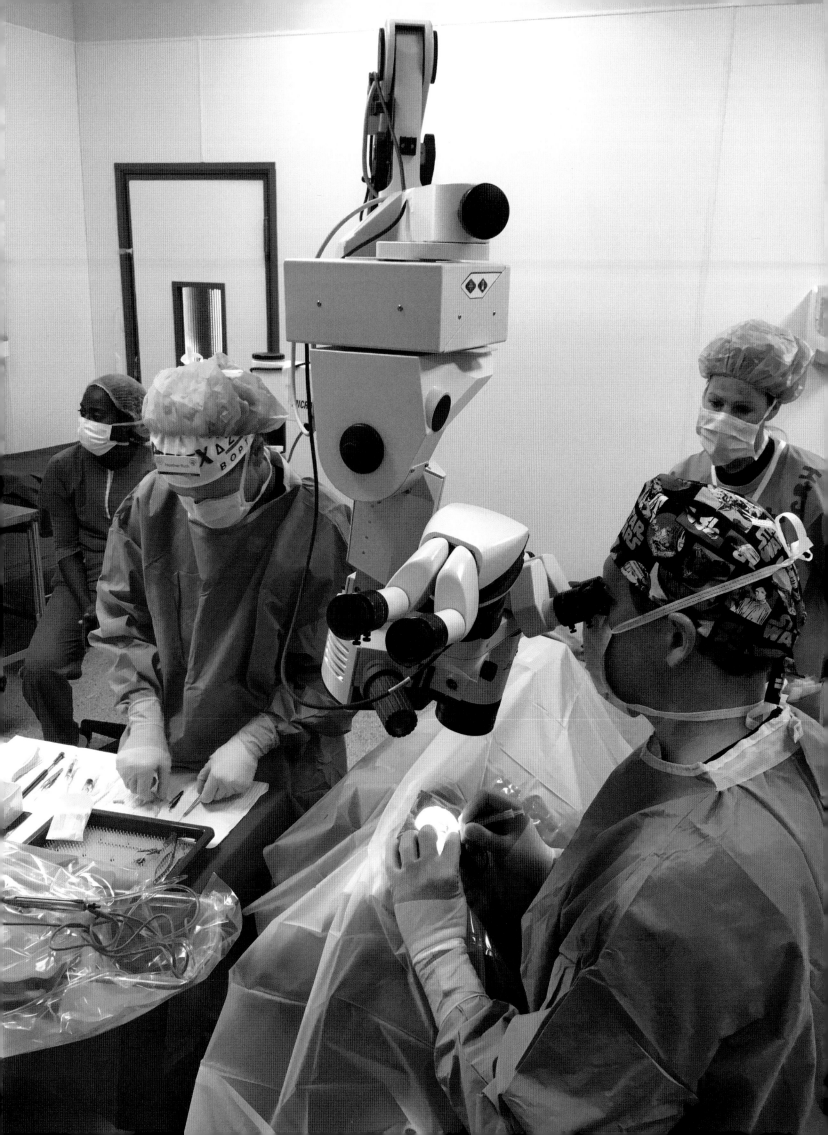

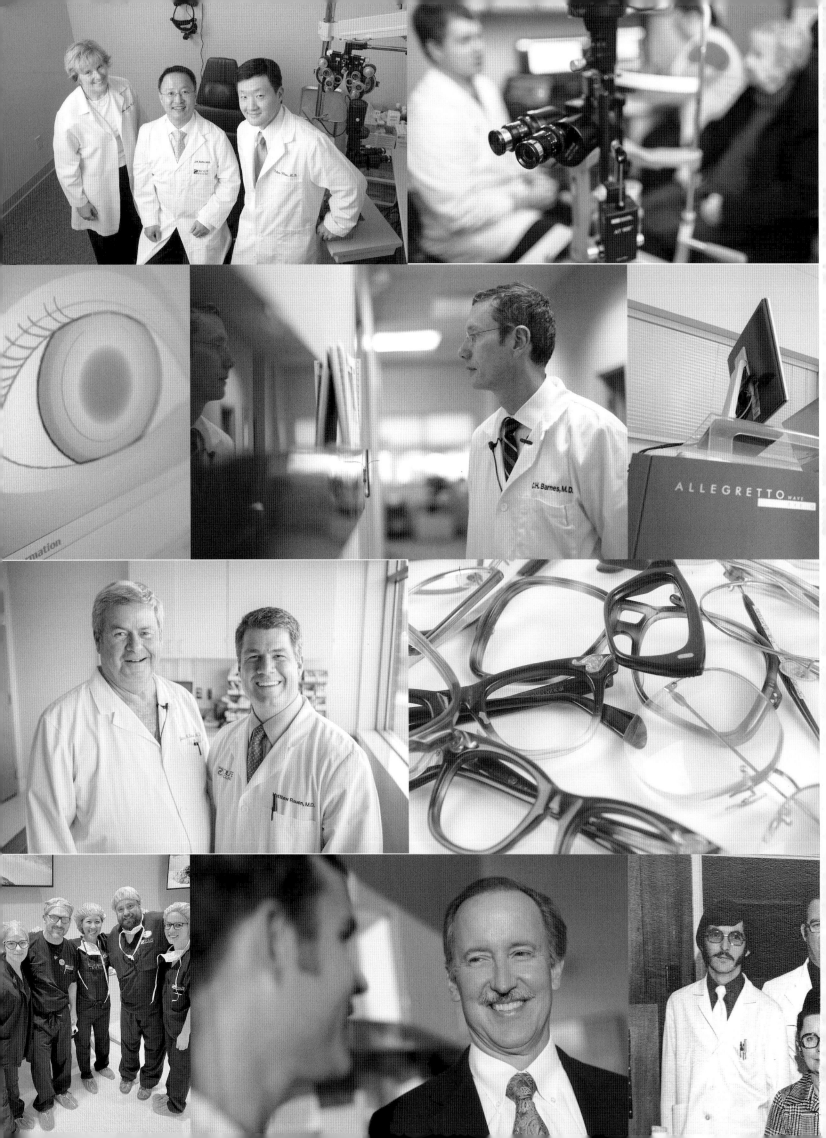